Glad to Be a Dad; Calm to Be a Mom

Written Specifically for Parents with Elementary-Aged Children

DAVID HOLDEN

ISBN 978-1-64258-211-6 (paperback)
ISBN 978-1-64258-212-3 (digital)

Christian Faith Publishing, Inc.
832 Park Avenue
Meadville, PA 16335
www.christianfaithpublishing.com

Scripture quotations are taken from the New International Version (NIV). All italics in the Bible texts were added by the author for emphasis.

Printed in the United States of America

To Caleb, Rebekah, Joshua, and Sarah who have taught me so much; and to Regina, my wife, who has given me time to learn

Hear, O Israel: The LORD our God, the LORD is one. Love the LORD your God with all your heart and with all your soul and with all your strength. These commandments that I give you today are to be upon your hearts. Impress them on your children. Talk about them when you sit at home and when you walk along the road, when you lie down and when you get up. Tie them as symbols on your hands and bind them on your foreheads. Write them on the doorframes of your houses and on your gates.

—Deuteronomy 6:4–9

But if anyone causes one of these little ones who believe in me to sin, it would be better for him to have a large millstone hung around his neck and to be drowned in the depths of the sea.

—Matthew 18:6

Fathers, do not exasperate your children; instead, bring them up in the training and instruction of the Lord.

—Ephesians 6:4

Fathers, do not embitter your children, or they will become discouraged.

—Colossians 3:21

But we were gentle among you, like a mother caring for her little children.

—First Thessalonians 2:7

May your father and mother be glad; may she who gave you birth rejoice.

—Proverbs 23:25

Contents

Preface

SOME GOALS ARE SO WORTHY; it's glorious even to fail. I can think of no greater honor and responsibility than to raise a child. I am not an expert at raising children; in fact, my college degrees are in business management (Biola University) and in Bible and Theology (San Jose Christian College). I have been married thirty years to my beautiful wife, Regina, and I am the father of four children, Caleb (26), Rebekah (24), Joshua (deceased), and Sarah (20).

My purpose for this book is simple: I want fathers to associate the joy they feel in being a dad with the joy our Heavenly Father feels in being our Abba Father. It is my observation that our earthly father–son relationship plays a significant role in our future Heavenly Father–adopted son relationship with God. A healthy relationship with our earthly father is not a requirement for a healthy relationship with our Heavenly Father; however, I believe it does play a powerful role in how we view, at least initially, our Heavenly Father.

I want mothers to associate the calm they feel in being a mom with the calm the disciples felt when they learned and understood Jesus could calm any storm on the sea with a single command. It is my observation that storms will come into every mom's life; however, God gives each mother this promise: "As a mother comforts her child, so will I comfort you" (Isa. 66:13).

God designed the family structure, and He chose to use this as an example of our relationship with Him. I have been working with school-aged youth for thirty-five years. The strongest Christian walks I have observed are usually found in the young people who have a quality relationship with their parents. The youth with the most mature Christian standing are not necessarily those being home schooled or those attending Christian schools; rather, they are those who meet with their parents as a family to read God's Word together; those who worship and serve together as a family; those who have real, authentic two-way dialogue about life; and those who pray regularly with their family members.

The love and affirmation children receive in the home are a direct linkage to a child's self-image and the way they respect other individuals. Parents too often expect youth programs and Christian schools to provide the primary instruction in God's Word for their children. *Read Deuteronomy chapter 6!* Parents are responsible for the training and discipline of their children. Youth programs and Christian schools are support networks to assist parents with this wonderful responsibility.

Coming back to my original intent: How awesome it is that God allows us to raise His children. Are our children any less loved by God than His own Son—Jesus—whom He revealed to the world as an innocent little baby, dependent upon his parents? *No!* Should we take raising our children any less seriously than Joseph and Mary did in raising Jesus? *No!* Will our Abba Father help us as He did Joseph and Mary? *Yes!*

In the pages that follow, I want to invite you to become excited about being a parent and to discover WHY God desires to use you. Learn how to become trans-*parent* with your children. Feel the joy our Heavenly Father expressed about Jesus on a high mountain we refer to as the Transfiguration: "This is my Son, whom I love; with Him I am well pleased. Listen to Him" (Matt. 17:5). May we develop this same joy and calm with our own children.

I could not publish this book without the consent, support and encouragement of my children – after all, they did most of the teaching. When I shared my opportunity to publish with them, their immediate response was to make sure that those who read this book understand that the Holden Family is flawed and often fell short. This is why the emphasis is upon WHY to parent, not HOW to parent. Perseverance and Passion for family are Regina and my primary parenting strengths.

I believe with all my heart that young parents today need to be encouraged and need to be reminded to enjoy the parenting process. I have included a devotional aspect to this book for those who want to use it as a personal devotional or in a parenting class setting. I asked my children, from oldest to youngest, to complete my preface for me. Their individual thoughts are recorded below.

Caleb: The saying, "hindsight is 20/20" is the perfect way to describe my view of how I was parented. Growing up, there were many times that my parents would do something (usually involving disciplining me) and I did not agree with their actions. However, it usually didn't take long for me to realize they were acting in the way they thought would best get my attention and help me become a better man. Now being in my mid-twenties, I can see why they parented the way they did and that they played a huge part in shaping me into the man I am today.

One of the things I love most about the relationship with my parents is that I have very different relationships with my mom and dad. I can talk to my dad about anything and we have a common love for sports that we love to indulge in together. My mom and I like the same type of movies and have a similar sense of humor. While we hung out a lot together as a family, my parents made sure that I had certain things I did with each of them, and they continue to embrace my different relationships with both of them.

In many parenting books, the author and their spouse can seem perfect. Our family was definitely not perfect because no family is. My parents made mistakes just like all parents do, as I'm sure to do once I become a parent. Though, what I appreciated is that when my parents would make a mistake, they would come apologize to me and ask for forgiveness. Having parents that owned up to their mistakes was one of the best models I could have had. It showed me that it's ok to mess up, but it's imperative that you acknowledge what you did and apologize. Overall, I have always had a good relationship with my parents because of the immense love they showed me; whether that was through words, actions, or discipline, they always showed me love and still do to this day. Having zero doubt that your parents love you and will run through a wall for you is one of the greatest gifts I could have ever asked for.

Rebekah: "To be loved but not known is comforting but superficial. To be known and not loved is our greatest fear. But to be fully known and truly loved is, well, a lot like being loved by God. It is what we need more than anything. It liberates us from pretense, humbles us out of our self-righteousness, and fortifies us for any difficulty life can throw at us." While this quote is from Timothy Keller's best-selling book on the Meaning of Marriage, I think the same applies to the deep and impactful relationship between a parent and child.

My name is Rebekah, and I am the middle child in our family of five. When my dad began writing this book many years ago, I remember how he would share about the joy and peace he felt in parenting, amidst the chaos and unpredictability of life. The older I get, the more grateful I am for the loving way my parents led our family. I can only hope that when God calls my husband and I to begin a family of our own, that we will follow in the example of making our kids feel known, cared for, and loved that my parents gave to me.

In reflecting back on my childhood, and the way my parents raised me, I am drawn to their characteristic of encouragement. More than anything, I never doubted that my parents believed in me. In moments where I would question my worth, identity, and future, my parents were always there to offer an encouraging word and cheer me on. They deeply valued time together as a family, and they instilled a true sense of belonging to the family of Christ, first and foremost.

While it would be easy to read this book with the lens that our family was perfect, what made us a supportive, healthy, and functional family was our imperfection. Each one of us kids had our own struggles we had to work through, and very much still stumble and fall, but we pick ourselves back up to this day. This healthy encouragement, provided by my parents, reminds me how it is often the imperfect moments where we are willing to vulnerably share our stories and courageously engage with those who mean the most to us. This is where we are given the opportunity to learn and grow together. As my dad shares in this book, there is great joy found in the journey.

Sarah: Mom and Dad, you both are an inspiration to me. Mom, I admire your kind, genuine heart. You have always been there for me and you have never judged me. I'm so thankful for the fact that I know no matter what, you will support me and be there for me. Dad, I greatly appreciate your wisdom and discernment. I never had to worry about anything because I knew you would always have my back. You've always made me feel so safe.

You both have showed me what I want my future family to look like. The way you love each other, and show love to us kids unconditionally, is incredible. I am probably the most thankful for the fact that you placed such a high emphasis and priority upon family time. Being best friends with your siblings isn't as common as it should be, but you taught us to rely on each other. Thanks to that, we have never, and will never, be alone. Being the youngest, I especially value the encouragement and support from you all. I love you so much.

Part I

Parenting Starts with a Healthy Marriage

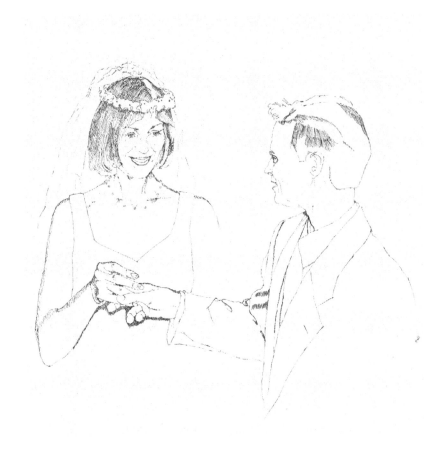

1

Marriage Requires…

Foundation

MATTHEW TELLS THE STORY OF two builders—one wise and one foolish (Matt. 7:24–27). Both men built houses that faced storms, but only the one with a solid foundation withstood the storm.

Marriage is a lot like these houses built upon sand and rock. The exterior may look great, but the underpinning is critical for survival. Like team sports, marriage requires commitment, teamwork, and a good game plan. The more solid the foundation of a marriage, the better the marriage responds to the storms of this life.

I will be the first to admit that many of the storms my wife and I face in our marriage are self-induced—pride, selfishness, stubbornness, conditional love, etc. Some of the storms we face are beyond our control and hit us at the weakest part of our foundation (Satan has good aim with his fiery darts).

However, whether our storms are self-induced or beyond our control is not the issue. Here is a fact: all marriages will face storms; therefore, a solid foundation is a must for continued survival! According to *The Future of the American Family* (Moody Press, 1993) and subsequent surveys by the Barna group in the mid-1990s, born-again Christians (27 percent) are slightly more likely than non-Christians (23 percent) to go through a divorce. Have these statistics changed any twenty years later? Sadly, No, according to Dr. Bradford Wilcox, Director of the National Marriage Project. While being interviewed in 2014 and responding to the question: "Are religious conservatives really divorcing more than religious liberals, or more than people who have no religious affiliation at all?" he states: "Yes." However, he gives some added detail that is extremely important to understand.

"Dr. Wilcox finds that active conservative Protestants who attend church regularly are actually 35% less likely to divorce than those who have no religious preferences. Nominal Christians, however, those who simply call themselves Christians but do not actively engage with the faith, are actually 20% more likely than the general population to get divorced." Perhaps there is a link between putting on a show in the religious and relational context versus true devotion to our Savior. Does consistent Church attendance as a family really make a difference? The statistics say they do. More importantly, I encourage you to ask parents and grandparents that you respect, in your church, if consistent Church attendance played a significantly positive role in their Marriage.

My personal observation finds the marriages best prepared to withstand life's storms are couples very actively involved in small groups and serving together as a family at church.

How can Divorce be so prevalent among professing believers? My belief is that Satan hates marital romance and will do everything he can to oppose it (domestic partnership) and to destroy it (divorce). Satan left God's kingdom because he wanted all the love and respect God was receiving for himself. Ephesians 5:25 states, "Each husband must *love* his wife as he loves himself, and the wife must *respect* her husband." In his twenty-year research project with couples, Dr. John Gottman from the University of Washington concluded that love and respect were the two primary ingredients for a healthy marriage. God knew this a little bit earlier. I believe a Christian marriage is an active player in spiritual warfare!

Do children influence a marriage? Do they create a need for change and flexibility? *Yes!* As children become a part of our new foundation, we must continue to build. This additional building must not stress the integrity of our current foundation or our house may collapse. In other words, do not build the children's wing on the sand. It sounds crazy to think that anyone would build a foundation made of rock and sand, but it happens. Believe me, Satan will find the sand in our foundation!

Similarly, we must be careful to not place such an emphasis on the children's wing that we allow the rest of the house to crumble from neglect. Translation: our marriage needs a strong foundation both before and after children; our children must never become our foundation, or divorce will conquer our marriage once the eaglets leave the nest.

My wife and I spent five years in courtship with one another, preparing a foundation that would last in marriage. The same commitment my wife and I needed from one another—to love, honor, and cherish till death do us part—is the same commitment our children need from us.

Dad, Mom, our children need to see our commitment to Christ; they need to see our commitment to each other; they need to see our commitment to them. All three are rudimentary for their future growth. When my oldest child, Caleb, was eighteen months old, he taught me this lesson: He wanted both his mother and his father together with him as much as possible. When I was at work, he spent the entire day with Mom and all he would talk about was Dad. When I was alone with him, he spent his time saying mama. When we were both home with him, he spent his time running back and forth between the two of us, often physically grabbing our fingers to bring us into the same room so we would all be together. Caleb needed to see his mother and his father together!

My youngest daughter, Sarah, at age ten asked me every night, as I tucked her into bed, what time would I be home from work the next day, and she suggested an activity we could do together as a family. Sarah was most content when the entire family was all together, especially if were watching her play softball, basketball, or soccer.

Fundamentals

IN THE MONTH OF MARCH each year, baseball teams gather in Arizona and Florida for spring training. The ballplayers practice bunting, covering bases, hitting their cutoff man—the fundamentals of the game of baseball. In the medical world, many hospitals require a doctor to assist in a surgery before actually performing it if he/she had not performed that specific operation over a given time period.

Why would professionals, who spent years learning how to perform, need a refresher course? Simple: it is our human nature to forget skills in which we once excelled. The moment we begin to think that we don't need to practice anymore is the moment we begin to regress. How long will a musician stay good if he stops practicing and playing his instrument? How long will a marriage stay good if one partner, or both, stops practicing the fundamentals of marriage?

Many words could be considered fundamental to a marriage; I have chosen four to look at.

Communication. This requires both time and effort. Most parents spend much time teaching their children how to talk but very little time teaching them how to listen. Communication requires both a sender and a receiver! Have you ever wondered why God gave us two ears and only one mouth? When we learn to be open and honest with our listening, as well as with our speech, we begin to truly communicate with one another. If you want to listen to a song on the radio, do you have the television on at the same time? If you want to actively listen to your spouse or child, should you have the television on at the same time? *No!* We allow too much outside static to infiltrate our receiving of communication. This is within our control.

Just listening is not enough. Speaking is only as good as it is open, honest, and truthful. Communication is only as good as it is framed in love. I know this is true for me: I need to think before I speak. What is my purpose in communicating this message to my wife? Guilt! Power! Control! Revenge! Manipulation! Do I want to resolve the conflict or do I want to win? Like an injured animal, when I hurt, I often want to strike back.

Refusing to speak can be just as deadly. My body language, which speaks very loudly in my marriage, can also do great damage. Direct, open, honest, truthful communication—framed in love, with a purpose of resolving conflict—spares many a battle. Recognize that every interaction with your spouse presents the opportunity to make a deposit or a withdrawal from the love/respect bank of their heart.

Husbands, become excited about telling your wife what you did today—they truly care; also, become excited about your wife's day. This will prepare you for becoming excited about listening to your children. Does your wife know that what she does with her day is important to you? How about your children, do they know you care about their day?

Our family tries to spend as many dinners as possible together at the dining room table (with the television and radio off and cell phones in a different room). We are developing the habit of sharing with and listening to each family member.

I encourage all wives to help their husbands communicate their feelings by asking the right questions (How did that make you feel?) and asking them at the right time (not the first minute he walks through the door or with two minutes left in any sporting contest). Does your husband feel appreciated and adored for all the hard work he does for his family? Ask him!

Trust. This is developed and strengthened over time. Trusting someone goes to the very core of our being since we are born into this world in such a helpless state. Christianity is based upon trust; we call it faith. Christians, by faith, believe that Jesus is the incarnate Christ, the God /Man who shed His blood at Calvary for our sins; that by this act of grace, we are reconciled to God and forgiven for our sins; and upon confession and acceptance of this act of grace, we receive an eternal inheritance and dwelling place with God.

Marriage is entered into as a trust relationship. Both partners pledge their lifetime devotion to one another, and they seal this trust with wedding rings. Each spouse trusts that regardless of any change (weight gain, paralysis, disease, money loss, etc.), the unconditional love of their mate will remain constant.

Lies, deception, and breaking of trust lead to deep hurt and immense pain. Broken trust can be healed over time—our Heavenly Father is the master healer, but living above reproach and never endangering that trust are the better ways to go. My wife and I have earned each other's trust—neither of us wants to do anything that would jeopardize our trust with each other. When children see the trust Mom has in Dad and Dad has in Mom, they will also soon develop that same trust in Dad and Mom. Are you trustworthy? Are you willing to become a model of trust for each child?

Forgiveness. This requires humility and courage. Forgiveness is another attribute grounded in Christianity. Our hope for eternal life with Jesus is based upon God's forgiveness of our sins. Does God take forgiveness seriously? Matthew 6:14–15 states, "For if you forgive men when they sin against you, your heavenly Father will also forgive you. But if you do not forgive men their sins, your Father will not forgive your sins."

Of course, forgiveness only applies after punishment has been rendered, restitution has been paid, and begging has commenced—*not!* Our sins are forgiven because Jesus suffered punishment, because Jesus purchased us for a price, and we need not feel guilty or beg. God's forgiveness is unconditional for all people at all times.

With this same unconditional acceptance and love, marriage is sustained by forgiveness. Let's face it, we all fail, we all err. Developing the ability to say "I'm sorry" is an absolute must for a healthy marriage. Receiving forgiveness without unneeded guilt or corporal punishment is refreshing. Giving forgiveness is soothing to our soul.

Husbands, do you love your wife enough to forgive her? Are you humble enough to realize that you err and hurt others from time to time and need to say, "I'm sorry"? Do you realize that your children will learn from you how to forgive and how to ask for forgiveness? Is your forgiveness unconditional like that of your Heavenly Father?

Wives, do you respect your husband enough to forgive him? Are you willing to pardon the hurt he has caused you?

Are you able to develop selective amnesia? Do you realize your children will learn from you how to absolve a hurt? Is your forgetfulness (as far as the East is from the West) like that of your Heavenly Father?

Love. This must be selfless and sacrificial. On my wedding day, one of my dear friends and groomsman (Howie) wrote and sang a song for my wife and me during our wedding ceremony. The chorus of that song follows: "Just remember to say I love you even if the love seems all gone, and remember to say I'm sorry when you've done the other wrong, but most of all remember to follow the Savior all the days of your lives. Then you'll have a love there's not many of. You'll have a love that will last you the rest of your lives."

Love is not a feeling that comes and goes like the blowing of the wind. Passion may be described that way, but not love. Love is one of the sections of the fruit of the Spirit that needs to be developed and nurtured throughout our lives. In 1 Corinthians 13:13, Paul reveals the three primary character qualities for a Christian to pursue—faith, hope, and love—but the greatest of these is love.

What is love? In the same chapter verses 4–7, Paul describes love as being patient, kind, rejoicing with the truth, always protecting, always trusting, always hoping, and always persevering. Paul continues by describing those actions which are contrary to love: being envious, boasting, pride, rudeness, seeking after self, becoming easily angered, keeping record of wrongs—not forgiving, and delighting in evil.

Our society teaches us to become our own person, to discover our higher self, to look out for number one, and to seek independence. The Bible, however, teaches that a married couple becomes one:

> Then the LORD God made a woman from the rib He had taken out of the man, and He brought her to the man. The man said, 'This is now bone of my bones and flesh of my flesh; she shall be called woman for she was taken out of man.' For this reason a man will leave his father and mother and be united to his wife, and they will become one flesh. (Gen. 2:23–24)

My wife, Regina, is not an added appendage that I can choose to ignore; she is not a grafted branch in a tree with many branches. She is flesh of my flesh and bone of my bone. This means that her concerns are my concerns; my joy becomes our joy; love for self becomes love for her. Giving my love to her is far superior than receiving my love from myself. God understood this when He decided to create male and female in His own image with a free will to love.

Husbands, do you love your wife as you do your own body, or do you treat her as an accessory whose main purpose is to make you look and feel good and to mother your children? Do you realize the sense of security your children feel when they see you selflessly and sacrificially loving your wife—their mom?

Wives, do you demonstrate your love for your husband by respecting his role as a servant leader? Are you careful to speak about him in positive terms in front of your children, extended family, and friends? Do you realize the sense of security your children feel when they see you support the leadership of your husband—their dad?

Never forget love is a choice! It is the choice that Jesus made in the garden of Gethsemane—He chose to die for you and me.

Companionship

THINK BACK ABOUT WHY YOU chose to get married. Was it for sex, money, or power? Most likely not! The number one reason why people marry is for companionship. We all want someone we know we can trust to love us and stay with us for the rest of our lives. It can become very lonely, for most people, to live by themselves. God gave Eve to Adam and walked with them in the garden of Eden (Gen. 3). Do you still go on consistent walks with your spouse and invite God to join you?

Companionship should be the result of two becoming one flesh. Song of Songs repeatedly states, "My lover is mine and I am his." We can't allow ourselves to become so busy with our vocation, or with our children, that we neglect our first calling: husband and wife. A husband and wife need at least two vacations of a couple nights duration—away from the children—each year to re-connect and recharge the romance and commitment to companionship—especially when the children are young. Your children need to see your commitment to one another.

I understand it can be difficult to schedule "couple" time away without the kids for many; however, difficult does not make it any less necessary. Find a way! Fly the grandparents in. Swap trips with friends from church. Share your children with parents at your church who no longer have young children to enjoy. Hire a responsible babysitter you trust to live at your house. Move closer to the grandparents or invite family to move closer to you. Even if the best you can do is to spend a night or two, half an hour away at a hotel—do it. Spending uninterrupted time alone romancing each other and relaxing together is always a very important part of a healthy marriage in every stage – especially the stage with young children. Make the effort! Believe it or not, God can ensure the safety of your children while the two of you are away for a couple of nights. Is your companionship a priority? Prove it!

I believe that the *foundation* protects and promotes a healthy marriage, the *fundamentals* sustain the marriage day in and day out, and the *companionship* keeps the marriage fresh and exciting. Can you think of any practical reason why a marriage must become stale? I'm changing; my wife is changing. What is stale about that? Many of the exciting marriages I have witnessed involve people who have been married twenty, thirty, forty, and fifty or more years.

If you are committed to loving your spouse and spending time with him/her, why not enjoy it? Develop common interests; discover what makes your spouse's eyes sparkle with joy—this does not always require great amounts of money to be spent. The gift of marriage is just that—*a gift from God.* If we are children of the king, we become a prince and a princess. Treat your wife as a princess. Treat your husband as a prince.

When Regina and I began our courtship process, we discussed frankly how we should view one another—as children of the King and as a gift—not to be opened without a covenant, a pledge, a vow binding us unto death. During our honeymoon, we opened our gifts and they are never to be returned.

Regina is my wife, the mother of my children and my best friend. Why would I not want to have fun with her? Freshness and excitement requires creativity and time spent alone—yes, this means finding childcare from time to time.

Husbands, your relationship with your wife will powerfully shape how your sons will view marriage in the future! Is it vibrant and fun? Or is it tedious and stale? Do you take time out to escape the stress of everyday life and remind your wife why you married her—for companionship! "The LORD God said, 'It is not good for the man to be alone. I will make a helper suitable for him'" (Gen. 2:18).

Wives, your relationship with your husband will powerfully shape how your daughters will view marriage in the future! Is it peaceful and romantic? Or is it tense and full of conflict? Do you take time out to escape the stress of everyday life and remind your husband why you married him—for companionship! "The wise woman builds her house, but with her own hands the foolish one tears hers down" (Prov. 14:1).

2

Life Hasn't Changed, Roles Have

A WHILE AGO, I ATTENDED my ten-year high school reunion and my five-year college reunion within several months of each other. This led to some inspection on my part to discover how much I have really changed. What I concluded was this: Life hasn't changed, my roles have. Below I will give four examples of this astonishing revelation.

Church

IN MY CHURCH, I HAVE gone from student to teacher, from being served to serving, and from receiving support to giving support (financial, emotional, and physical). My church is still a church—a meeting place for those who desire to worship God and learn more about Him and His Word. It is my role in the church that has changed!

Going to church was something I did every Sunday with my family. I was often a spectator and observer. As I have grownup and matured, I have discovered that church is much more than mere observation. It is the vital foundation of God's kingdom that is being established and used by

God for His glory through His people. As God has blessed, equipped, and prepared me, I have moved from a passive role to an active role.

My Sunday mornings and evenings are still being spent at the same location; however, the way in which I spend them is different because my role is different. My role is different because my knowledge and understanding of church is different. As our knowledge and understanding increases, so must our roles. *God chooses to use us!* James 1:22 says it better: "Do not merely listen to the word, and so deceive yourselves. Do what it says." First Corinthians 13:11 states, "When I was a child, I talked like a child, I thought like a child, I reasoned like a child. When I became a man, I put childish ways behind me."

As our faith, hope, and love increase—as Jesus becomes more eminent in our life—our roles must change from one who is served to one who serves, from one who receives to one who gives. Our Heavenly Father will equip and promote us as we are willing to be changed. God is calling us to become servant leaders!

Family leadership is foundational for church leadership. First Timothy chapter three describes qualifications for choosing church leaders. Verses 4 and 5 state, "He must manage his own family well and see that his children obey him with proper respect" (if anyone does not know how to manage his own family, how can he take care of God's church?).

Rather than separate church from family, we must learn to use fusion—uniting together, blending into one! What is a church? A church is fellow believers uniting together to further a common purpose (for Christians, that purpose is to *increase God's kingdom* through evangelism, discipleship, and fellowship; to *actively worship God*—Father, Son, and Holy Spirit; and to *love and respect* God's creation—people and planet). Love God, love people and help others do the same!

What an awesome family ministry we can have together! Imagine the closeness a family will develop as they seek to increase God's kingdom, actively worship God, and love and respect His creation together as a family. Parents, don't wait for your child's youth pastor to teach the importance of missions or the intimacy of worship or the need to love people or the beauty of creation to your child. You take the initiative! Plan family outings and vacations with these things in mind.

One of the most wonderful experiences of my life was baptizing each of my children in our church, on Palm Sunday, when they were seven years old. I am not a pastor. I am not a church officer. I am simply a dad who was honored and overjoyed to help my children follow Jesus' commandment to be baptized.

Our family should imitate a small church. Mom/Dad, you become the Shepherd and follow the words of Proverbs 27:23, "Be sure you know the condition of your flocks, give careful attention to your herds." Serve the Living God together as a family. The Philippian jailer and his entire family came to know God after a violent earthquake released Paul and Silas from prison. Acts 16:34 records these words: "The jailer brought them into his house and set a meal before them, he was filled with joy because he had come to believe in God—he and his whole family."

Consider the house of Cornelius where the apostle Peter learned that salvation was for the Gentile as well as for the Jew. Acts 10:2 states, "He and all his family were devout and God-fearing; he gave generously to those in need and prayed to God regularly."

Parents, teach your children how to give—allow them to experience serving in a food and clothing shelter (our family has served together at the local Salvation Army). Allow them to help choose how and where to send financial gifts—adopt a child through Compassion International or World Vision or International Justice Ministries, contribute money to Focus on the Family, deliver supplies to local or church missionaries. Allow them to visit hospitalized patients or senior citizens to spread hope and to learn compassion.

My daughter, Rebekah, has visited at least five countries on mission trips before her 25th birthday. For her 16th birthday she decided she wanted to spend the day serving at a local rescue mission in our city. She called her friends and family, set-up the day of service and even found a way to organize a worship service that had me preaching and her leading worship. She had a wonderful junior high youth pastor, Justin, and high school pastors, Will and Dave, and parents who taught her that she could change the world at a young age. Was it easy as a parent to send her off to Africa and Central America as a teen-ager to serve and tell others about Jesus? Honestly, No! But it was necessary – she belongs to Him!

As church and family become one, we become a community. Church becomes less of a place and more of a lifestyle, religion gives way to relationship, and serving God becomes an everyday event, rather than a once a week occurrence.

Family

IN MY FAMILY, I HAVE gone from son to husband, from child to father. I still have the same parents. I still have my same brother; however, my emphasis, my responsibilities {my role} have changed. I am no longer expected to just show up on time for dinner; I am now expected to help provide and help prepare dinner. I don't need to ask for the keys to the car or have to be in by curfew; I now hope there is a car and fall asleep before curfew!

I am still in a family—an extended family with in-laws—but the roles of husband and father are very different from my role as eldest son. I enjoyed being the eldest of two sons. I love having a younger brother who is still my good friend. My point is simple: as I left my Mother and Father and cleaved unto my wife, my responsibilities have changed; my roles have changed. I greatly enjoyed being a son—and still do—but I also greatly enjoy being a husband and a father.

Identity is a key issue here. If my identity is in what I do for a living (businessman) rather than in whom I am (a husband and a father), I will make foolish life decisions by prioritizing my work over my family. Follow my reasoning for a moment: I could stop being a businessman by being fired or by choosing a different profession. Can I be fired from being a husband or a father? Can I choose to stop being a husband or a father? Unfortunately, divorce has made this possible. We treat who we are—our identity—the same way we treat what we do. Too many husbands and fathers today view these roles as just another job description alongside their profession.

Many moms work outside the home or inside the home as telecommuters today. Some moms are the primary wage earner for the family and Dad stays at home with the children. Some moms "home school" their children full-time each day, while other moms provide child care in their home. This same struggle for identity hits mom. Dads need to understand this!

The enemy is attempting to, and often times succeeding at, making us so busy, we lose sight of our primary objective: to enjoy our relationships with God and with one another. When we lose our joy, the Bible says we lose our strength; when we lose our strength, we lose our witness. Exodus 18 gives a wonderful story of how Moses was so busy serving God as judge for the people, he did not have time for his own wife and two sons. Moses's father-in-law, Jethro, came to Moses and in verses 17 and 18 told Moses, "What you are doing is not good. You and these people who come to you will only wear yourselves out. The work is too heavy for you; you cannot handle it alone." He taught Moses how to delegate and administrate so Moses would have time to spend with his family.

As parents, we need to teach our children the benefits of working together as a family. Some children, like my daughters Rebekah and Sarah, will love to help clean the house. Other children, like my son Caleb, will battle his parents all day long when it comes to helping clean the house (boys need to learn household chores and dads need to help lead by example). Our children learn valuable lessons in teamwork and responsibility, and the rewards and consequences associated with them, when we, as parents, include our children with housework assignments.

My wife has been offered incredible wages to do after school care of neighborhood children. The extra money would be wonderful. The temptation to say yes is very strong. For some families, yes may be the correct answer. For our family, we have chosen to say no because my wife's primary purpose for staying home is to care for, teach, and love our children. Although the extra income would be beneficial, the sacrifices of time and spontaneity are greater than the benefits of the extra income.

If you are a spouse and/or a parent, I challenge you to view this as your highest calling from God. What is God's will for your life? To love your spouse and children with all your heart, soul, and mind and to help them in their daily walk with Jesus. Anything else—building a church as a pastor, being a dentist, being a doctor, being a lawyer, being a soldier—must become secondary. Your relationships here on earth are eternal—your profession is temporary!

Matthew 6:19–21 states, "Do not store up for yourselves treasures on earth, where moth and rust destroy, and where thieves break in and steal. But store up for yourselves treasures in heaven, where moth and rust do not destroy, and where thieves do not break in and steal. For where your treasure is, there your heart will be also."

What do you treasure most? Is it your relationship with your spouse and child(ren)? Or is it the prestige you receive from your job? What ladder are you attempting to climb? The one in your corporate or social structure? Or the one to your family's heart? This may mean saying *no* to a promotion. This may mean changing your current employment. This may mean moving your family to a more affordable location (many of our young family friends moved out of state so Mom could stay home). God will honor those who honor Him! Choose that which is eternal over that which is temporal. Below are the words to a song entitled "Slow Down" by Michael James.

Well, you've worked late every night this week
You went in early today
You think that if you're to climb to the top
That's the price you've got to pay

You haven't had supper with your kids all week
There's more work than ever before
Guess you didn't hear what your oldest child said
This morning as you walked out the door

Slow down, Daddy, don't work so hard
We're proud of our car; we've got a big enough yard
Slow down, Daddy, we want you around
Daddy, please slow down

Matthew hit his first home run last night
Daddy, you'd have been so proud

After the game when we all went to bed
Thought I heard Momma crying out loud

Your job is important, we all understand
We're thankful for all that you do
But nothing can replace the happiness
That we have when we're with you

Slow down, Daddy, don't work so hard
We're proud of our car; we've got a big enough yard
Slow down, Daddy, we want you around
Daddy, please slow down

Work

AT MY JOB, I HAVE gone from employee to manager; from one who is told what to do to one who does the telling; from one who punches a time clock to one who wishes he could punch a time clock and be paid overtime. I have worked for the same employer since I was seven (7) years old (my father owns a company that provides personnel dosimetry service—Radiation Detection Company), so my workplace has not changed. However, my role with the company has changed dramatically!

When I was seven years old, my father would pay me less than minimum wage for performing simple work functions at home. That was not enough! I negotiated a pack of baseball cards for every half hour worked or the deal was off. Several years later, I negotiated the same deal for my brother. The money I earned was of course spent on more baseball cards. Life was so simple!

I spent my high school and college summers at the work place (more money, fewer baseball cards) and was very fortunate to develop a good sense for business and a strong work ethic. The company offered me a full-time job upon graduation from college with a degree in business management, which I accepted. Since college, I have worked my way up from employee to supervisor to manager to vice president.

I realize that my work history is uncommon, but the pressure to succeed and to provide for my family is common. With each successive promotion, I made it clear to my employer that time spent with my family is more important to me than additional money or prestige. I am very fortunate to be working for a company that recognizes the importance of family.

I am not suggesting that Christian workers should not seek to grow and gain more responsibility; I am suggesting the contrary—our business world needs men and women with integrity, men and women with ethics, men and women who value what God values.

What we need is a balance! I have worked my share of Saturdays. I have called during a meeting and told my wife I couldn't make it home in time for dinner. What I have not done is to allow this behavior to become the norm rather than the exception. My family understands that my work is important and helps put food on the table; my family also understands that they are more valuable to me than my job. My strong desire to spend time with my family only makes me a better businessman. I strive to become efficient with my work time in order to avoid unneeded extra hours at the office because I was lazy or chewing the fat.

The pressure to provide for my family financially and still be able to spend time with my wife and my children is very real. Throw in my time spent serving at church, seeing friends and family, and of course doing yard work and various house chores, and the hours of each day get shorter and the money in my wallet gets thinner. I understand! Regina stopped working, outside the home, after she gave birth to our firstborn. Suddenly, our budget became paycheck to paycheck; I felt pressure to work longer and harder to make ends meet. What is the solution?

The solution is simple: work hard and serve well and focus on that which is eternal!

Therefore I tell you, do not worry about your life, what you will eat or drink; or about your body, what you will wear. Is not life more important than food, and the body more important than clothes?…And why do you worry about clothes? See how the lilies of the field grow. They do not labor or spin. Yet I tell you that not even Solomon in all his splendor was dressed like one of these… So do not worry, saying, "What shall we eat?" or "What shall we drink?" or "What shall we wear?" For the pagans run after all these things and your heavenly Father knows that you need them. *But seek first His kingdom and His righteousness, and all these things will be given to you as well.* Therefore do not worry about tomorrow, for tomorrow will worry about itself. Each day has enough trouble of its own. (Matt. 6:25–34; emphasis added)

Is simple faith a solution? Or is it an excuse for not trying? The pressure parents face is real—we can't just stop working and spend every moment with our spouse and child(ren); however, a child's need for dedicated family time spent together is also real.

Fathers, how much money is worth missing your child's ballgame? Is a vacation home worth more than watching your child laugh as you play with him or her? Is that nice car for you or for your family?

Mothers, how much discretionary income is worth missing your child's first word? First step? First tooth? Who is teaching your children how to discern what they watch with their eyes? What they hear with their ears? What they speak with their mouth?

Please allow me a sidebar for one moment: we must be sensitive to economic reality. Most single mothers have zero alternatives to working outside of the home. The same can be said for many traditional two-parent families (especially those living in the Bay Area, California). The questions to ponder for these families are different, albeit along the same line of reasoning.

Consider working thirty hours outside the home rather than forty hours so you can be home for the kids after school (many employers offer benefits at thirty hours per week). Consider employment inside the home—the digital age has made this a very practical alternative for some. Consider job sharing with another mom. For some families, having Mom work outside of the home and Dad watching the child(ren) may make more economic sense. I would caution that this scenario should only be used when *Mom wants* to work outside of the home.

Thanks for the sidebar. What do I propose? When we are able to, we (parents) need to choose time spent with our family and trust God to honor that commitment. This will require sacrifice! Look at the budget—maybe by driving a less expensive car or by eating out less often or by becoming more efficient with our time, we can relieve some of the pressure we feel.

If Jesus is our ultimate model—*and He must be*—read the four Gospels and see how much time He spent with His children (the twelve apostles). Parents, if we choose to place our family first, if we choose to trust God to provide, and if we choose to love as He first loved us, we will be successful in our calling—to love our spouse and to raise our child(ren) in the training and instruction of the Lord.

School

IN SCHOOL, I HAVE GONE from a shy elementary school student to an adjunct teacher of graduate students. From one who had to go to school to one who chooses to go to school. Things have not changed much, I am still in school; however, my motivation for school has changed. From elementary school through high school, I had one goal in mind—get to the next highest level and one day it would all be over.

Going to college was the first time I really felt like I had a choice in whether or not I would attend school. When I researched the difference in job responsibility and job pay between a high school and college graduate, I no longer felt like I had a choice. I entered college with one goal in mind—to graduate and enter the "real world." I discovered that the real world was different from college, but not necessarily any more difficult nor more rewarding. I look back with some regret for not enjoying my college experience more. Too often I chose books over people.

After working full-time as a businessman for two years, I began to feel complacent and in need of a further challenge. So I decided to go back to school—this time because I really wanted to. The challenge began: working full-time while taking three college classes. Then along came Caleb. The ultimate challenge began: working full-time, taking classes, and helping raise a newborn. How easy it would have been to give up my goal of a bachelor's degree in Bible and Theology. I had to work and help raise the newborn; going to school was just a choice. *Wrong!*

Going back to school was more than just a choice—it is a lifestyle! I believe that too many of us think we reach an imaginary point where we no longer need to be a student. We sit back in the pew on Sunday morning and tune out the message because we have heard one like it before or maybe even taught it before. We don't have time to read books. We have already read through the entire Bible four times during our lifetime—nothing new happens that we don't already know.

This self-proclaimed arrival is very dangerous! When we stop studying and learning, we start deteriorating. This does not mean that we have to enroll back in school—which is what I chose to do. It does mean that we must always hunger for spiritual knowledge and thirst for understanding. Hebrews 5:13–14 states (emphasis added), "Anyone who lives on milk, being still an infant, is not acquainted with the teaching about righteousness. But solid food is for the mature, *who by constant use* have trained themselves to distinguish good from evil."

Jesus adds in John 7:37–38, "If anyone is thirsty, let him come to me and drink. Whoever believes in me, as the Scripture has said, streams of living water will flow from within him." We must remain teachable so the Holy Spirit can mold us and teach us how to best love and represent Christ.

What kind of medical doctor no longer looks at his medical journals because he already read it twice? What kind of lawyer refuses to keep studying the law and case history because he has passed his bar? Some of our evange-lism and discipleship programs that worked so well in the 1980s may not work today in the 21st Century. Who would choose a personal computer made in the 1980s over one made today?

The point of this discussion is really quite simple: we must never stop learning, never grow complacent, and never believe that we have arrived. How can we encourage our children to study and learn if we refuse to do the same?

If you want your child to enjoy learning, participate in the learning process with him/her. Don't throw up your hands and blame the school system; rather, step up and fill in the gaps that exist in our educational system. The best way to communicate the importance of learning about Jesus to your child(ren) is for them to see you continuing to learn—to see you excited, even after all these years, about reading the Word of God and about hearing it preached.

Why did I go back to school? To learn more about Jesus, the One whom I serve. My friends and coworkers had trouble understanding that. They felt for sure that I must be headed for church ministry or the mission field.

Why did I not quit when Caleb was born? Because learning is too important to quit. I made other adjustments instead—less softball tournaments, fewer nights out with friends, decrease in number of units I was taking, less time spent watching sports on television, etc. Sacrifices had to be made. We must learn to sacrifice the correct things—they do not include family time, church time, or learning time.

Let's consider parenting! Where do we go to school to learn how to parent? When you carefully chose your vocation, you likely took school classes to prepare you for your new job. You likely participated in numerous hours of "on-the-job" training. You likely have received more hours of training for new procedures and new duties. Why? So you can confidently and efficiently perform your job. Why not apply the same standard to parenting?

God has equipped us with a natural parenting intuition (especially mom) and has given us the Holy Spirit and His Word to help us along the way. If your supervisor on the first day of your new job told you to use your natural intuition and this procedure manual to get the job done and left you alone, how successful would you be?

God wants us to learn! Our natural intuition to parent, God's Word, and the guidance we receive from the Holy Spirit are priceless. God has given many of us parents and grandparents to help teach us. He has given us a church family to support us. He has given some of us close friends and/or mentors with parenting experience to assist us. He has given us many wonderful books on parenting (I hope this becomes one of them).

The church I attend, First Baptist Georgetown – in Texas – does a wonderful job of encouraging our young parents to continue learning by providing wonderful opportunities. Parents can take their children to AWANA, or youth group programs midweek, and attend encouraging marriage and parenting classes while the children attend their program. Young parents are provided mature mentors who come to their home to offer counsel and encouragement. Junior High and High School parents are encouraged to attend Sunday morning small groups where they study and discuss the lesson plan for the upcoming Wednesday night with the youth pastor. Parenting resources are provided, family serving opportunities are given and young families know they are cared for and supported in the great adventure of parenting.

Mom and Dad, I want to encourage you to study and prepare for a lifetime of parenting and then pass along your wisdom to your children when you become a grandparent. Take notes, try new techniques, remember your successful moments, and forgive your failures. Enjoy the learning process. Each child is very different, and they each deserve the best parenting you are capable of giving to them.

Grandparents should be encouraged to have healthy, supportive, loving relationships with each grandchild. Our children were fortunate to live close by all of their Grandparents. Grandparents were the first to take a grandchild on a motorcycle ride, horseback ride or to Spring Training in Arizona. They attended hundreds of ballgames, established Christmas traditions, organized and paid for family vacations and dozens of dinners out, provided shoulders to cry on, encouraged spiritual growth, spent hours praying and built family memories that will last for eternity. To this day in their twenties, our children's grandparents remain very active in each of their lives and these relationships are precious and powerful.

Learning can take place in many different ways. Studying or attending classes and seminars is one way. We can also learn through our experience. This may include field trips, volunteer work, or direct observation. The most important question in the learning process is who is doing the teaching?

> We have not received the spirit of the world but the Spirit who is from God, that we may understand what God has freely given us. This is what we speak, not in words taught us by human wisdom but in words taught by the Spirit, expressing spiritual truths in spiritual words. The man without the Spirit does not accept the things that come from the Spirit of God, for they are foolishness to him, and he cannot understand them, because they are spiritually discerned. The spiritual man makes judgments about all things, but he himself is not subject to any man's judgment. (1 Cor. 2:12–15)

The Holy Spirit, who indwells believers, must become our primary teacher. Learning is a lifelong process when the Spirit of the Living God becomes our instructor. Parents, we must continue to learn so that we will be properly equipped and able to teach and train our family in the way of righteousness. How exciting it is to learn about the goodness of God *together* as a family! Below are the words to a poem, which sits above my desk at home, entitled "The little chap who follows me," written by an unknown author who obviously understood that parents become teachers.

A careful man I ought to be;
A little fellow follows me;
I do not dare to go astray
For fear he'll go the self-same way.

I must not madly step aside,
Where pleasures paths are smooth and wide,
And join in wine's red revelry—
A little fellow follows me.

I cannot once escape his eyes:
What're he sees me do he tries—
Like me, he says, he's going to be;
The little chap who follows me.

He thinks that I am good and fine,
Believes in every word of mine;
The base in me he must not see,
The little chap who follows me.

I must remember as I go,
Through summer's sun and winter's snow,
I'm building for the years to be,
A little fellow follows me.

3

Divorce from a Kid's Perspective

Another thing you do: You flood the Lord's altar with
tears. You weep and wail because He no longer pays
attention to your offerings or accepts them with pleasure
from your hands. You ask, "Why?" It is because the Lord
is acting as the witness between you and the wife of your
youth, because you have broken faith with her, though
she is your partner, the wife of your marriage covenant.
Has not the Lord made them one? In flesh and spirit
they are His. And why one? *Because He was seeking
godly offspring.* So guard yourself in your spirit, and
do not break faith with the wife of your youth.
"I hate divorce," says the Lord God of Israel, "and
I hate a man's covering himself with violence as well
as with his garment," says the Lord Almighty.
So guard yourself in your spirit, and do not break faith.
—Malachi 2:13–16 (emphasis added)

To the married I give this command (not I, but the
Lord): A wife must not separate from her husband…
And a husband must not divorce his wife.

To the rest I say this (I, not the LORD): If any brother
has a wife who is not a believer and she is willing
to live with him, he must not divorce her. And if a
woman has a husband who is not a believer and he
is willing to live with her, she must not divorce him.
For the unbelieving husband has been sanctified
through his wife, and the unbelieving wife has been
sanctified through her believing husband. *Otherwise
your children would be unclean, but as it is, they are holy.*
—1 Cor. 7:10–14 (emphasis added)

YOU PROBABLY HAVE HEARD OR read about the damage a
divorce can do to the adults involved. You may have experienced this damage yourself. The best analogy I have seen
is of two pieces of paper, which have been glued together
for years, being separated. Neither piece of paper will
escape undamaged, and the change will be permanent.
Each piece of paper contains miniscule pieces and fibers
from the other because they truly had become "one" piece
of paper.

At the same time, we must recognize that divorce is
not the unpardonable sin. Through God's forgiveness and
healing, that takes place over time, a divorced person can
develop healthy relationships and overcome the hurt and
pain they have experienced.

I am ashamed at how insensitive some Christians are
to divorced men and women. Of all the people who need
to experience the love of Jesus, people who have recently
been divorced are toward the top. Remember, God commands us to love.

Still, God hates divorce. I understand that at times marriage can be very difficult (broken trust, substance abuse, emotional abuse); however, I believe that obtaining legal help from our court system and counseling help from a qualified counselor is the better solution. Being equally yoked and marrying a spouse *because* of their walk with Jesus is the best solution.

Scripture contains some great examples of "tough marriages" (God with spiritual Israel and Hosea with Gomer), and the overlying principle is one of faithfulness, patience, perseverance, and love. Many divorces, however, are not for abusive reasons. The reasons are varied and often the result of irritability, incompatibility, perceived irreconcilable differences, and the belief that "I can do better" or "I will be happier if…"

Whatever the reason may be, children are too often overlooked when divorce is chosen. Being a child from a divorced home, I would like to speak about divorce from the "kid's" perspective.

On their twenty-fifth wedding anniversary, my parents began the official court process of ending their marriage. I was twenty-three years old and had just returned from my honeymoon when my mother treated me to lunch and announced the news of the pending divorce. I wasn't shocked because I was aware of their stormy relationship over the last ten years. The timing was bad, but the foundation had been crumbling for years.

The divorce was in no way amicable, and both my mother and my father tried hard to explain the reasons why and conjure up support for their position. Fortunately, my brother and I knew that both contributed to the downfall of their marriage, so we tried hard to listen without passing judgment. The settlement took nearly two years to conclude.

I had to endure the unfortunate experience of being employed at the same family-owned business that both of my parents worked for. The first six months, I saw my mother and my father every day at work. Imagine, here I am the Human Resources Manager with sixty employees under my management; my father (president and owner of the company) had just moved out of a nice house and into a small one-bedroom apartment; my mother, who worked at home for twenty-five years, was now coming into work. It was my job to interface with each of them on a daily basis. I became the primary vessel of communication. I had to deal with it!

When I look back on those first six months, I remember a lot of frustration, anger, hurt, and resentment. I also remember God's peace that surpasses all understanding. I am grateful for friends who listened to me and allowed me to express my pain without telling me I was wrong to feel that way. I appreciated my friends not broaching the subject until I brought it up. I was blessed to have in-laws who proved to me that marriage can last—and be good! My pain was abundant; however, God's comfort was even more abundant.

After the first six months, my feelings came under control, my mother found a new job, and my pain was replaced by excitement for my own marriage, which continued to hum despite my time of despair. I am very glad that I took the time to mourn my parents' failed marriage. A death truly took place in my life. I felt cleansed and my relationship with my risen Savior moved to a new level of dependency.

My experience is familiar for many people. Divorcing parents often have great compassion for their children during the first six to twelve months of a divorce. But life must go on, right? Yes, but life has changed permanently! Both of my parents remarried within two years of the start of their divorce. For the most part, their past is dead and gone. They started a new life and want to look forward; the past is too painful to remember.

For my brother and I, however, the past is full of great memories of growing up with Mom and Dad—vacations, ballgames, and family night—but whom can we share these memories with? I don't want my past to die—it is part of who I am today!

Divorce is painful for everyone involved during the first year. Today, three decades later, my parents' divorce causes more problems for my brother and me than for either of them. My parents are both genuinely content in their new lives. They endured great pain and still bear some of the scars today, but for the most part, life is good.

My brother and I are left with dealing with the challenges. Do we talk about the past? Where do we go for the holidays? Who do we invite to each party or event? How can we spend some quality time alone with Mom or Dad without offending their spouse? How do we get Mom and Dad to open up with us and remain an active part of our life?

The parent–child relationship is built upon trust. Communicating with my parents was always very easy for me. Now, because of a breach of trust between my parents, my relationship with each parent became hampered. Somehow, because I was linked to "the other," the trust and depth of conversation I once knew were no longer available. I felt like I kept hitting a brick wall whenever I tried to deepen the level of conversation with either parent. The scars they bear from the hurt they endured kept them from risking a deeper level of vulnerability. Worse yet, they did not recognize this.

Trust builds with time, and I eventually rebuilt that deeper level of communication. My love for my parents allowed me to persevere; however, how many children are willing to make this effort? My brother and I were adults, twenty-one and twenty-three, respectively, when we had to deal with these issues. How do two brothers, eleven and thirteen, handle these same situations? How do two sisters, five and seven, handle these same situations?

My brother and I had a firm faith and reliance upon God to help see us through; we had a support system of mature friends already developed and in place. We still struggle with some of the issues we face today; painful feelings still resurface from time to time. How do children deal with this?

The answer is quite frightening! Children often respond with rebellion, fantasy escape, blaming of self, refusal to communicate, unhealthy relationships to discover lost love, substance abuse to numb the pain, or by joining a group to gain acceptance (gang, sports team, cult). The reason is quite simple. The child's basic need for a "sense of belonging" has been destroyed before his/her very eyes. Children gain their identity from their parents. When characters are first introduced in scripture, the majority are introduced as the "son of..."

I wanted my parents to accept and love me so my actions were determined accordingly. From my earliest thought, I understood that I needed my parents to survive—a natural trust develops on the part of the child.

Destroy the marriage. Destroy the identity! This is where my brother and I were fortunate—our identity was with *Jesus Christ*! Little children haven't made this correlation yet. Many children never do! They become sucked up by their pain and confusion.

Children of divorced parents need a solid church youth group; divorced parents need a solid Bible-based support group. I pray that our churches today will accept and reach out to these families—the world certainly will!

Husbands and wives, if you are considering a divorce, please reconsider. Consider speaking rather than silence, forgiveness rather than vengeance, and persevering rather than quitting. Seek godly counseling. Pray for guidance from the Holy Spirit. All marriages go through rough waters. If we keep our life jacket (*faith*) on and never stop paddling (*works*), God can see us through and our marriage will become even stronger. Perseverance breeds strength. "We know that suffering produces perseverance; perseverance, character; and character, hope. And hope does not disappoint us, because God has poured out His love into our hearts by the Holy Spirit, whom He has given us" (Rom. 5:3–5).

Please do not decide to "tough it out" alone for the sake of the children. This will often lead to resentment, and it will only postpone the divorce. The time to deal with marital problems is as they occur—don't wait. Growing up as a child in a family that constantly views Mom and Dad fighting, or refusing to communicate, is not healthy either. The child's trust will never fully develop, and confusion and doubt will consume them. Whom do I identify with, Mom or Dad? Whom do I attempt to please? Why would I ever want to get married?

Regardless of the ages of your children, a divorce is going to hurt, and negative consequences will result. Children need to see Mom and Dad in love with one another and serving Jesus together. No marriage is beyond repair—for in Christ Jesus, all things are possible. Heed these words from Jesus in Matthew 18:5–6: "And whoever welcomes a little child like this in my name welcomes me. But if anyone causes one of these little ones who believe in me to sin, it would be better for him to have a large millstone hung around his neck and to be drowned in the depths of the sea."

If you are reading this and are already divorced, or if you are an unwed mother or father, please know that God loves you and still has plans of hope for your future. Like the woman caught in adultery and brought to Jesus, God is more interested in building your future than in judging your past. Choose to be a loving parent and release all feelings of guilt and shame at the cross. Glad to be a dad? Calm to be a mom? It begins with being happy to be a husband and joyous to be a wife!

Part II

Little Lessons I'm Learning

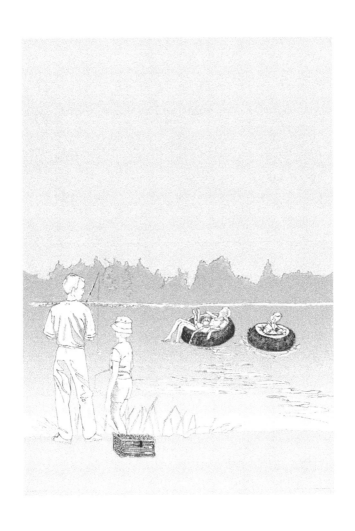

4

Self-Control

PROVERBS 25:28 DESCRIBES MY YOUNGEST daughter (Sarah) when she was eighteen months old perfectly: "Like a city whose walls are broken down is a man who lacks self-control." I am not talking about outright rebellion or even purposeful sinning here. I am referring to the inability to say *no* to anything that looks fun, exciting, and risky!

At eighteen months of age, my daughter did not weigh out her options; she did not consider the consequences of her actions; she did not think before she acted. She simply coveted and responded accordingly!

The desire that catches her eye ignites a spark of passion in her little heart and she goes for it! She reminds me of the fish that smells the bait. Sometimes, like the fish, she gets away with the bait; however, more times than not, she swallows the bait—hook, line, and sinker—and winds up in the hands of the fisherman!

I don't refer to this "catch" as sin—it is more of a natural curiosity. The telephone makes such neat noises when the buttons are pressed. Mom's hair provides comfort when it's yanked and cuddled. Little rocks taste so good. The garbage can is full of so many surprises. Teeth naturally come together on Dad's skin when she becomes excited. Books look better on the floor than on the shelf.

The first couple of times these infractions occurred (thirteen to fifteen months), the response was natural and without guilt or fear. Guess what? As Mom and Dad disciplined little Sarah, ignorance gave way to understanding; disobedience gave way to obedience. As a two-year-old, Sarah still struggled with the above behaviors, but she had developed the capacity to overcome her desire—she learned to say *no* to enticement.

Sarah would often point to the books or phone or garbage can and say no as she pointed to it. Guess what? Her struggle shifted to times when Mom and Dad were not present.

Her young understanding allowed her to conclude that if Mom and Dad don't see her do it, she can't get caught. She quickly learned that this reasoning is faulty. To summarize: my daughter learned what is acceptable behavior by what she was taught; she learned self-control through discipline, and she learned that eyes are always upon her.

Sarah's big brother and sister committed the same actions as a two-year-old (Mom and Dad are much better prepared the third time around). As they grew up, our preteen children still struggled with phones, rocks, and books (the phone was answered without permission; rocks were tossed all over the grass instead of in the mouth; books were lost, found, and lost again), but their *understanding* of acceptable behavior and their *ability* to control their actions had matured greatly.

This study in human nature became painfully familiar to me as a representation of my relationship with God. God has given me His Word to communicate what is acceptable behavior for me as His child and what is not acceptable behavior. "All scripture is God-breathed and is useful for teaching, rebuking, correcting and training in righteousness, so that the man of God may be thoroughly equipped for every good work" (2 Tim. 3:16–17).

God also dwells within me (Holy Spirit), setting up residence in my body (His temple) and reminding me daily of my commitment to obedience. "Do you not know that your body is a temple of the Holy Spirit, who is in you, whom you have received from God? You are not your own" (1 Cor. 6:19).

Despite these constant reminders, I still allow myself to become enticed by the world around me. "For everything in the world—the cravings of sinful man, the lust of his eyes and the boasting of what he has and does—comes not from the Father but from the world" (1 John 2:16).

God's response to my disobedience, like my response to my daughter's disobedience, is discipline encased with love. "Endure hardship as discipline; God is treating you as sons. For what son is not disciplined by his father?… God disciplines us for our good that we may share in His holiness. No discipline seems pleasant at the time, but painful. Later on, however, it produces a harvest of righteousness and peace for those who have been trained by it" (Heb. 12:7–11).

As I become more aware of my struggle areas, my weaknesses, I begin to say *no* in public, but, too often, I still say *yes* in private. Just like my daughter, I do not get away with anything either. God is omniscient (all-knowing) and omnipresent (ever-present). The decision is mine to make. I now have the ability to control my desires and say *no* to unrighteousness and *yes* to godliness. How? By becoming filled with the Spirit of God and allowing Him to develop the fruit of self-control in my life.

> His divine power has given us everything we need for life and godliness through our knowledge of Him who called us by His own glory and goodness. Through these He has given us His very great and precious promises so that through them you may participate in the divine nature *and escape the corruption in the world caused by evil desires.*
>
> For this very reason, make every effort to add to your faith goodness; and to goodness, knowledge; and to knowledge, self-control; and to self-control, perseverance; and to perseverance, godliness; and to godliness, brotherly kindness; and to brotherly kindness, love. *For if you possess these qualities in increasing measure,* they will keep you from being ineffective and unproductive in your knowledge of our Lord Jesus Christ. (2 Pet. 1:3–9; emphasis added)

My daughter's struggle with desire as a two-year-old is a reflection of my struggle with desire as an adult. I pray that my response to her will be as loving and as helpful as my Heavenly Father's response is toward me. I thank God that as a father, I can learn *how* to discipline, *how* to forgive, *how* to instruct, *how* to love my daughter, and *how* to assist her through these struggles, by listening to and learning from *how* God nurtures me.

The more self-control I develop in my life, the more self-control I can help my daughter develop in her life. Listen during your prayer time with God today. You will hear Him praise you for the choice of self-control you made rather than giving in to that sinful desire you were tempted by. Our children need to hear this positive praise from the lips of their earthly parents as well. Catch your children doing things right!

God has given me His Word to communicate what is acceptable behavior and what is not acceptable behavior.

5

Incarnation

WHEN MY SON CALEB WAS eleven months old and beginning to crawl around very well, I experienced a stunning
revelation on the incarnation of Jesus Christ. Normal for
his age, Caleb had a very short attention span—reminds
me of some adults I know—as he crawled around from toy
to toy, from object to object, and from person to person.

One day while I was playing with him, I noticed that
whatever object I began to play with, he wanted to play
with. When I would pick up a ball and begin to toss it
around, he would gaze at me for minutes (this is a long
time for a little guy) as though I had invented the greatest
toy on earth. I could see him trying to figure out how that
same ball, which is so out of control in his hands, obeys my
every wish. Without fail, he would come take the ball out
of my hands and try to do the same thing. He couldn't, but
that did not seem to matter. He was modeling his father's
behavior and that was joyful enough.

As I picked up the next toy, the same process occurred.
Caleb watches; Caleb laughs; Caleb models my behavior;
Caleb laughs. This modeling of my behavior continued

from age eleven months on through his preteen years. The objects changed from toys to equipment and from playing games to learning skills, but the process of following my actions was still the same.

The lesson is simple, words are rarely exchanged—he sees my behavior and he attempts to model it. I believe Jesus Christ came to earth as a man for us to view His behavior and then attempt to model it. Sure, we always fail to do as well as He did, but the longer we try, the more mature we become and the better we get at imitating Him.

Yes, Jesus did come to earth to die for mankind's sins; however, if that was the only purpose for His coming, He could have come for only three years or three months or three days and accomplished the same thing. He came as a helpless, dependent infant so we could watch and imitate.

After washing the disciple's feet, shortly before He was put to death, Jesus' words are recorded in John 13:15 as follows: "I have set you an example that you should do as I have done for you." The Gospels record three and one-half years of Jesus' ministry so that we—His children and followers—may watch and imitate.

The word *disciple* simply means "one who follows." In Matthew 16:24, Jesus says to His disciples (followers): "If anyone would come after me, he must deny himself and take up his cross and follow me." Jesus expected people to follow and imitate Him while He was here physically on earth, and He expects the same today. He lived a perfect life and demonstrated to all mankind the depth and width and height of God's love for us.

The only way mankind could relate to Jesus Christ and want to follow Him was if He came to earth in the same way we all do—birth as a baby. If He came as an adult, we would say that he avoided being "messed up" by those teenage years. If He came as a teenager, we would say that he avoided being "messed up" by those infant years. We can all understand the fears and joys of entering the world as a child, living as a teenager, and becoming an adult. We can relate to Jesus because He can relate to us!

> Since the children have flesh and blood, He too shared in their humanity so that by His death He might destroy him who holds the power of death—that is, the devil—and free those who all their lives were held in slavery by their fear of death…For this reason He had to be made like His brothers in every way, in order that He might become a merciful and faithful high priest in service to God, and that He might make atonement for the sins of the people. Because He Himself suffered when He was tempted, He is able to help those who are being tempted." (Heb. 2:14–18)

When I became aware of my son's intent to follow me, a scripture verse written by Paul leapt into my mind. In 1 Corinthians 11:1, Paul tells the Corinthian believers, "Follow my example, as I follow the example of Christ."

Parents, are we willing to say this to our children today? Am I willing to tell my son that if he listens to my words and watches my actions, he will learn about Jesus? *Yes, I am!*

I will explain to him that I am not perfect and that I all too often miss the mark (sin), but I will not let the fear of failure keep me from trying to be a godly example to my son. When I err, I will ask for forgiveness and help him understand where I went wrong. When I fail to do the good I should have done, I will help him understand why I allowed fear to stop me. When my attitude sucks, I will identify the cause and correct it. Whether my sin is one of commission, omission, or disposition, I will try my best to overcome it and correct any wrong I may have done.

I believe that parents need to become servant leaders for their children. The world provides many role models displaying its values. Our children need to know that we are willing to risk our pride, to risk potential failure, and to risk leaving our comfort zone so that they may have an example to follow—one that leads to eternal life with Christ Jesus. Parents, we all too often expect our children's teachers or coaches or the pastor of our church to provide this model for us—it is our responsibility!

If we are unwilling, our children will look elsewhere. Today is the day to start, do not wait until they are in junior high school or high school. My son started imitating my actions naturally at eleven months old. Until he is able to comprehend what it means to be a disciple of Jesus Christ, I want to continue to be the one that he chooses to imitate.

The joy in my son's face when he successfully imitated my actions serves as a constant reminder to me that great joy can be found in following Jesus. The apostle Paul tells Timothy in 1 Timothy 6:6, "Godliness with contentment is great gain." What a great goal to have: to be godly, to be content, and to introduce my son to Jesus.

I learned another lesson about the incarnation of Christ from my eleven-month-old son. When we were in the same room together, he would cry out for me. He would crawl around my feet and let me know that he wanted something. I could not sit in the same room or walk into the same room without him becoming upset; however, the moment I picked him up or sat down on the floor, he was ecstatic. The light bulb turned on!

Caleb simply wanted to be on the same level with me. It did not matter if I brought him to my level or if I joined him on the floor at his level. He simply wanted us to be on the same level. He wanted to feel my touch. For intimacy to take place, for bonding to take place, two people need to be on the same level with each other. I am talking about the same eye level. About walking in the same shoes.

Jesus came to earth as a man to join us at our level—so we could understand Him rather than drown in confusion. So we could relate to Him rather than fear Him. Our relationship with Jesus can be intimate because He meets us at our level! From the moment God first created mankind (in the garden) to leading His people into the promised land (through Moses and Joshua) to sending His one and only son to redeem us (salvation) to His imminent return for us (when Jesus comes again), God has always met us at our level.

Mom and Dad, are we willing to meet our children at their level—to remove confusion and fear thus opening the way for understanding and love—to lead us into an intimate relationship with our children? The incarnation of Jesus is all this and more, and I thank my son for helping me discover that.

Jesus came to earth as a man to join us at our level – so we could relate to Him rather than fear Him.

6

Security and Trust

I HAVE FOUND THAT MY greatest sense of security stems from trust. The greater my trust, the greater my belief, the greater my faith—the more peace and security I experience. I believe this is a universal truth: as trust increases, so does security increase. The opposite is true as well: as trust decreases, so does security decrease.

Children are born into this world with a natural sense of trust; unfortunately, by the time adulthood rolls around, many people have little to trust and consequently have very little security to hold on to.

In order to meet this security need in our life, we turn to religion, relationships, or other "things." "Things" can come and go—so will security. Religion is empty and quickly gets old—good-bye security. Relationships can last and can provide security that lasts; relationships can also fail and can bruise an individual so deep that trust never resurfaces again in one's lifetime.

I believe firmly that a relationship with Jesus Christ is the only relationship that will provide constant peace and security without fail. Other relationships, such as marriage, friendship and parent/child, can provide security, but the security provided would neither be constant nor consistent.

How much security can a relationship with God give? Hear the words of King David in Psalm 17:6–9 (emphasis added):

> I call on you, O God, for you will answer me; give ear to me and hear my prayer. Show the wonder of your great love, you who save by your right hand those who take refuge in you from their foes. *Keep me as the apple of your eye; hide me in the shadow of your wings* from the wicked who assail me, from my mortal enemies who surround me.

Hear the words of the author of Hebrews in Hebrews 6:17–20 (emphasis added):

> Because God wanted to make the unchanging nature of His purpose very clear to the heirs of what was promised, He confirmed it with an oath. God did this so that, by two unchangeable things in which it is impossible for God to lie, we who have fled to take hold of the hope offered to us may be greatly encouraged. *We have this hope as an anchor for the soul, firm and secure.* It enters the inner sanctu-

ary behind the curtain, where Jesus, who went before us, has entered on our behalf.

Hear the words of Paul in Romans 15:13 (emphasis added):

> May the God of hope fill you with all joy and peace *as you trust in Him,* so that you may overflow with hope by the power of the Holy Spirit.

I stated earlier that children are born into this world with a natural sense of trust. They are extremely dependent upon their parents for survival and they have no past hurts to make them distrust. During her preschool age, my oldest daughter (Rebekah) had no fear whenever her daddy was nearby. She walked off steps into my arms because she knew that I would catch her (this happened whether I was paying attention or not); she leapt into my arms into the swimming pool; she screamed for joy whenever I swung her around in circles; she jumped on my back for piggy-back rides. She had no concept of fear whenever she was in her daddy's arms.

Rebekah felt secure! If she fell and injured herself, she would run into my arms or into the waiting arms of her mother. She loved to hug and just be held. She had security needs! Every night before she went to bed, she would listen to me sing "you are my princess" and would respond with a giant hug and kiss. She knew her daddy would protect her while she slept.

Parents also have security needs. Sure, our children usually express these needs more often than we (parents) do, but our security needs are just as real and are just as important.

I believe God refers to us as His children for a good reason. We spend the first twenty-five years of our lives striving for independence, learning to trust in our own skills and abilities for survival; however, the Bible instructs us to "trust in the LORD with all your heart and lean not on your own understanding; in all your ways acknowledge Him, and He will make your paths straight" (Prov. 3:5–6).

In 2 Chronicles, chapter 20, we are told a beautiful story of trust. King Jehoshaphat was leading Judah and was on the verge of being attacked by Edom, who was vast and very powerful. King Jehoshaphat called all the families of Judah together to pray before the Lord—concluding his prayer in verse 12 by saying: "For we have no power to face this vast army that is attacking us. We do not know what to do, but our eyes are upon you." Verse 13 states: "All the men of Judah, with their wives and children and little ones, stood there before the Lord."

What a beautiful picture of faith and trust and godly leadership. God's response in verses 15–17 is even better: "Do not be afraid or discouraged because of this vast army. For the battle is not yours, but God's ... You will not have to fight this battle. Take up your positions; stand firm and see the deliverance the Lord will give you." As families, they entered the battlefield singing praise songs to the Lord and when they arrived they found nothing but dead bodies lying on the ground.

This same God loves and protects His families today. When we face the storms of life, our job as parents is to gather together our family, placing our eyes upon Him, allowing God to go before us. We need to model this for our children, so they model it for our grandchildren.

We should be striving for dependence instead of independence. Dependence upon Jesus; reliance upon the leadership of the Holy Spirit; trust in the LORD! It is so good to know that when I step out in faith, God is here to catch me; when I fall down and get hurt or when I am afraid, God is here to hold me. When I am tired, God is here to rock me and give me nourishment.

I felt so much joy whenever Rebekah came to me for a hug or wanted to be held or needed to be rocked in my chair. I enjoyed seeing the sense of security she felt whenever I was near. I believe that God feels that same joy when we come near to Him. He created us, He died for us, and He sustains us. We need to learn to let go of our problems and fears, and fall into His strong, loving arms unafraid. As Parents, we need to be careful to not make our children too dependent upon us. Our calling is to help them transition from dependence upon us to dependence upon Jesus. Sometimes, in our aim to protect them, or in our selfish want to keep them close to us, we stifle their growth by refusing to encourage them to transform (see Romans 12:2).

I have watched very well intentioned, loving parents hinder and impede the social growth of their children due to fear and/or selfishness. The goal of parenting is to raise godly children who are dependent upon Jesus and who are able to leave the home and make an impact upon this world for Christ by the end of high school. Our aim is to produce responsible children, who are able to confront and tackle life's problems and dilemmas with maturity and good sense – utilizing Biblical convictions and relying upon the Holy Spirit to give them direction.

We must allow our children to experience failure at a young age, while we as parents are here to help pick them up and encourage them to try again. As a mother Eagle drops her Eaglets out of the nest from the crest of the mountain to teach them how to fly, we as parents need to facilitate growth with our children by encouraging them to learn how to ride a bike (and later how to drive a car), how to save and spend money, how to make and keep friends, how to study, how to listen, how to learn, how to keep a promise and how to dream and pursue their passions. If Mama Eagle does not initiate the growth, some of her Eaglets will be content to never learn how to fly.

I get it! I loved being the most interesting, exciting and important person in my children's life, and I loved trying my best to meet their every need. It made me feel important and needed. But for their sake of maturity, I needed to allow them to make new friends; to become part of teams and youth groups that I did not coach or lead; to allow other teachers to instruct them; to allow godly adults to take them away for a week or longer to church camp or mission trips. My children have all attended mission trips (without their parents) since sixth grade and it continues today in college and beyond (and to other Continents). They coach, they teach, they mentor and they lead – because they had godly people in those capacities in their lives that invested in them and now they want to pay it back.

Was it easy to let go? Heck No! But it is absolutely necessary if I want them to transition from my voice and my convictions to God's voice and His convictions. Did I stay very actively involved in listening to what they were being taught and help them process conflicting values and beliefs? Absolutely Yes! I praise God for the godly leaders in their lives who taught them they were never too young to be used by God. Thank you, Will, Justin, Brad, Dave, Austin, Scott, Jimbo, Brett, Kendall, Tanya, Deanna, Moni, Chenney and Amy.

Fathers, are you aware of the importance of trust in your relationships with your wife and children? Do they see you as one who is dependable, reliable, and approachable? Are you willing to be the one in whom your children can trust and find security? Are you willing to point them to the ultimate source of peace, contentment, and security—a personal relationship with Jesus Christ—the only one who will never fail them? Are you willing to demonstrate and live out this trust yourself?

Mothers, do you realize the security, balance, and order you provide to your children and to your husband (many husbands have a hard time verbalizing this reality) by being at home when they return from the world? Being welcomed home with soft eyes and open arms provides a comfort beyond description. Mom, if you can financially afford to be home for the arrival of your children from school and for your husband from work, do it! An enthusiastic, loving greeting will set the stage for the rest of the evening.

Save the confrontations/discussions for later. With your actions, remind your family that "home" is a welcomed and safe rest place from the world in which we live. Mom, are you making sure your family views coming home as a rest haven away from chaos, strife, and tension? Does your family view home as a place of security and trust?

Parents, if you answered yes to your questions above, you will experience the joy our Heavenly Father experiences when His children come to Him—the cleft in the rock, the hiding place, the ever present help in times of trouble. The parable of the lost Son (Luke 15:11–32) demonstrates to us that even on our worst day, God welcomes us home with affection and excitement.

Parents, if you answered no to your questions above, your children may turn to other relationships, other religions, or "things" to fill their need for security. Or they may decide that no one and nothing can be trusted and live a life full of insecurity.

If home is just as stressful and negative as the world, why come home? This question applies for our spouse as well. We need to turn our house (building where people live) into a home (a safe dwelling place for family members, full of love and encouragement and joy). Sounds a little bit like heaven!

Choose today to be the example. Establish Jesus as your security and the basis for your trust. Build a solid marriage with your spouse. Develop a secure relationship with your children.

7

Love

AFTER A STRESSFUL DAY AT work, I knew that I could depend on three people to cheer me up—my children. As soon as I walked through our front door, they always, without fail, came running over to hug me with huge smiles on their faces. This is unconditional love and acceptance. It didn't matter what went on all day, the love of my children greeted me as I walked through that door. Unfortunately, this stage did not last forever, but I sure did enjoy it. For some strange reason, greeting Mom and Dad at the door became a lower priority once the "double digit" years hit.

What kind of love do believers receive when they meet with Jesus any time, any place, anywhere? *Unconditional love and acceptance!* And this is not just a stage, it lasts forever. This does not mean that our sins do not carry natural consequences—they do; however, forgiveness is only as far away as confession. "If we confess our sins, He is faithful and just and will forgive us our sins and purify us from all unrighteousness" (1 John 1:9).

Do you ever wonder why Scripture so often refers to mankind as *children of God*? "How great is the love the

Father has lavished on us, that we should be called children of God! And that is what we are!" (1 John 3:1). The words of Jesus recorded in Matthew 18:3 states, "I tell you the truth, unless you change and become like little children, you will never enter the kingdom of heaven."

Little children are known for being dependent, full of joy, being quick to trust and slow to judge, and for their unconditional love and acceptance. Why is it that we can place little children of all race, gender, socioeconomic status, religion, and creed in the middle of a grass lawn with a ball and watch them play unhindered for hours, but we can rarely bring together this same group of adults anywhere—church included—without a disruption soon occurring? The answer: children are quick to accept others while adults choose to judge and tolerate or despise.

What is it that occurs during our formative years that changes us from loving others to tolerance or indifference, from acceptance to dislike, and from trust to fear? The answer is *sin*! We live in a world full of sin. The world teaches us to look after our own needs over the needs of others, to hold the right of choice over the right to life, to avenge rather than to forgive, to have discord rather than unity, to put on masks rather than to be authentic, and to fear those not like us rather than to appreciate our differences.

These are all *learned behaviors*, contrary to the natural inclinations of a baby. A baby chooses to love because he hasn't yet learned to hate; a baby chooses acceptance because he hasn't yet learned to reject; a baby chooses to trust, to believe, and to hope because he hasn't yet learned to deceive, to disclaim, or to despair. We need to learn again how to love!

Scripture is full of examples of unconditional love (the father of the prodigal son, Jesus on the cross, Jesus with the woman caught in the act of adultery, Hosea and Gomer). The most quoted verse of Scripture (John 3:16) begins with "For God so loved the world…," an entire chapter (1 Cor. 13) is devoted to the importance of love, and an entire book (Song of Songs) is devoted to the expression of love. My favorite passage on love is the one my wife and I had read during our marriage ceremony.

> Dear friends, let us love one another, for love comes from God. Everyone who loves has been born of God and knows God. Whoever does not love does not know God, because *God is love.* This is how God showed His love among us: He sent His one and only Son into the world that we might live through Him. This is love: not that we loved God, but that He loved us and sent His Son as an atoning sacrifice for our sins. Dear friends, since God so loved us, we also ought to love one another. No one has ever seen God; but if we love one another, God lives in us and His love is made complete in us. (1 John 4:7–12; emphasis added)

Love is listed as the first of the nine sections of the fruit of the Spirit in Galatians 5:22–23. For fruit to become ripe and ready for consumption, a tree must be planted in good soil and take up firm root, be watered for nourishment, and pruned for sustained growth. Love is a fruit! We must decide to plant it in good soil. Next, we must allow the Holy Spirit to water for nourishment and prune for sustained growth. One more thing I have noticed about fruit—it spoils if it is not consumed. Like fruit, our love needs to be tasted by everyone we come into contact with; otherwise, it will spoil and be useless. And one spoiled fruit will spoil an entire barrel of fruit if not removed. Let your love become ripe and share it with others.

When I observed my daughter, Rebekah, day in and day out, I saw love. I saw her love for people, her love for interaction, her love for life. Her love was not biased, her love was not prejudged, her love was not impure or deceitful; her love was unconditional and full of acceptance. My daughter's love more closely resembled the love of Jesus than my love does.

One day, Rebekah (at age four) was eating an "otter pop" with her friend Michael in our kitchen. Michael dropped his otter pop, it spilled onto the floor, and he began to cry. Rebekah immediately gave her friend her otter pop and began cleaning up the mess. No "tough luck," "bad break," or "be more careful next time" was uttered. Just an unmerited gift to wipe away the tears. A great example of God's grace given to us.

One way Regina and I chose to show love to our children was through celebration. Throughout Scripture, God encouraged the Israelites to remember/honor the memory of significant events. This often resulted in a celebratory

feast or the building of a monument—so the next generation would remember God's favor.

We need to celebrate our children's significant milestones and accomplishments. Keep it simple. Make it
memorable. After a good report card, we went out for ice
cream. Birthdays generated a special family dinner on a
special birthday plate—and later a full-blown sleepover
with friends. Baptisms were cheered. Holidays meant parties with friends and family—simply reminiscing about
old memories, while creating new ones, and always playing games. Our family still celebrates together today, just
minus the sleepovers.

A very significant tradition our family embraced
involved our elementary-aged children graduating to
become teenagers. We found a two-mile hiking path that
ended in a park. Three mentors (pastors, grandparents,
teachers, parents) who spoke into their young lives waited
at each half mile. I walked the emergent teen into the
woods telling them how proud I was of them and offering
sage advice.

After one-fourth mile, I hugged them, shared Proverbs
3:5–6 with them and told them to follow the path. One-
fourth mile down the road, they met mentor #1, who
offered counsel and passed them on to mentor #2. Mentor
#1 followed behind with me. The process ended with men-
tor #3 walking them into the park—where all the child's
family and friends awaited them with buckets of chicken
or pizza to celebrate this milestone.

The party ended with everyone in a circle and the child
in the middle. Everyone was given the opportunity to share

a story and word of encouragement for the new teen. We ended with a giant huddle prayer for the child. Afterwards, the child was presented with a notebook containing a one-page note of encouragement and godly advice from parents they knew and loved (Mom began collecting and organizing these notes months in advance). Our children were encouraged to keep this notebook and to look back through it whenever they needed encouragement.

Heading off to college was a similar format involving mentors at a dinner (at a nice restaurant) presenting them with notes and encouraging words. Many of these celebratory ideas come from a book entitled *Raising a Modern-Day Knight*. I found this resource (along with many other wonderful parenting resources and family videos) at Focus on the Family (a Christian organization I wholeheartedly support and endorse). Celebrating milestones with friends and family made our children feel loved and important and reminded them they are "surrounded by a great cloud of witnesses" (Heb. 12:1).

Parents, learn from your child(ren) how to love. See the joy that accompanies such love; feel the peace that results from such love; experience the freedom and forgiveness that flows from such love. Relationships built upon unconditional love and acceptance will stand the storm like the house built upon the rock. Relationships built upon anything else will fall during storms like the house built upon the sand.

Mom and Dad, our children must know that our love will not decrease when they fail or do wrong; they must have the freedom to experience failure without the pressure of conditional love. Do we treat our child to a lunch at In-N-Out Burger if he/she gets two hits in the baseball/softball game but take him/her straight home if he/she goes 0–4? Do we reward our children for getting A's but not for B's? What if they give their best effort and receive a B? These examples may sound trivial, but they speak volumes to our children.

Conditional love teaches our children that results are more important than effort; that the end justifies the means; and that what we do is more important than who we are! These are fallacious beliefs that stem from conditional love. Character is more important than accomplishments! God—our Heavenly Father—does not love us because of what we have done; rather, He loves us because of who we are—His children. We can learn much about love by watching our child(ren).

We must allow the Holy Spirit to water for nourishment and prune for sustained growth.

8

Image

Then God said, "Let us make man *in our image*, in our
likeness, and let them rule over the fish of the sea and
the birds of the air, over the livestock, over all the earth,
and over all the creatures that move along the ground."
So God created *man in His own image*, in the *image of
God* He created him; male and female He created them.
—Genesis 1:26–27 (emphasis added)

When God created man, He made him in the likeness of
God. He created them male and female and blessed them.
And when they were created, He called them "man."
When Adam had lived 130 years, he had a son in his
own likeness, *in his own image*; and he named him Seth.
—Genesis 5:1–3 (emphasis added)

WHAT DOES IT MEAN TO be in one's image? To be in one's
likeness? Following are some facts for your consideration!

Mankind alone is created in the image of God.
Mankind is the climax of God's creation.

Mankind is still in the image of God after the fall.
The image of God upon mankind infers a special dignity.
The image of God gives mankind the
right to exercise dominion.
Male and female are both created in the image of God.
Man in his totality is in the image of God.
Man is made for relationship with God.
Man is made to function in God's image.

To be in one's image goes much deeper than physical resemblance. It is man as man (body, soul, and spirit) that is the image of God. This special dignity denotes worth and acceptance from the One whom creates. Our Heavenly Father could not give us, His children, any greater worth than to be created in His image! We are created in the image of the Perfect, Holy, and Loving, Awesome God!

In order to help us understand the essence of this reality, God allows us to bear and raise children in our own image, in our own likeness. How many children would be aborted if mankind realized they were aborting the very image of God?

In Genesis chapter 9, God explains to Noah that mankind is still in the image of God (after the fall) and that his blood is not to be shed. Although sin did not remove the image of God from mankind, it did create some competition against the image of God.

Mankind revealed a sinful nature that competes against the spiritual nature. The spiritual nature comes from the Holy Spirit indwelling born-again believers. Our spiritual nature desires for us to display the image of God for His glory. Our sinful nature desires for us to hide the image of God in the vain attempt to receive self-glorification.

The extent to which we display the image of God in our life is the extent to which we become conformed to the image of Christ. Second Corinthians 3:18 (emphasis added) explains it this way: "And we, who with unveiled faces all reflect the Lord's glory, are being *transformed into His likeness* with ever-increasing glory, which comes from the Lord, who is the Spirit."

The image of God is like the wings of a butterfly. Our sinful nature wants us to crawl around like a caterpillar—never realizing the potential we have to fly, to be free, to display God's glory. Guess what? God provides a cocoon in the person of His very own son—Jesus Christ—who will turn all who believe into butterflies. As we realize the image of the one whom we belong to, we stop crawling and we start flying! How does this relate to our children? Let us return to the facts about being in one's image.

Our children alone are created in our likeness.
Our children are the climax of God's creation.
Our children remain in our image, even after they fall.
Our image infers a special dignity to our children.
Our children are made for relationship with us.

My son, Caleb, is created in my image. His eighteen-month-old picture compared to my eighteen-month-old picture is remarkably similar. By age ten, he was already showing leadership and organizational skills that I possess. He was also showing an excessive amount of energy and stubbornness that I also have. I am amazed at how much of me I see in him!

He not only had these natural qualities within him, but he tried to be like me in every endeavor. He laughed when I laughed; he sang when I sang; he wanted to eat when I ate (he even ate his hamburgers plain with only a tomato like me); he followed me around from room to room. I became increasingly aware of the role model I would play in his life.

A perfect example occurred one night during dinner. Caleb, at twenty-two months of age, held out his hands and said "pray" when we sat down to eat dinner. We tried to always include him in saying grace before we ate; however, until that night, we were not sure if he had any clue as to what we were doing.

It is very convenient for parents to conclude that, at a young age, our children do not recognize violence on television, arguments in our marriage, anger or bitterness in our hearts, or inconsistent behavior in our lives; however, I quickly learned that my son, before he even turned two years of age, clearly recognized all of the above.

My heart leapt for joy the night I saw Caleb extend his hands toward me to say grace. Parents, the effort is worth it. It may take a while for the correct response to follow, but please do not give up. If I call my wife a jerk and storm out of the room, what will keep my children from calling their mother a jerk and storming out of the room? If it works for Dad…On the flip side, if a child sees his dad kissing his mom and telling her how much he loves her, he/she will be more likely to respect Mom and demonstrate love toward her.

Children learn through observation. They see an action and they decide to repeat it. If they receive a favorable response—laughter, praise, and a smile—they will continue the behavior. If they receive the dreaded *no*, they will either stop the behavior or try it again with the hope of soliciting a different response. *Your child is never too young to observe!*

Parents, do you treat your children as the pinnacle of your life—as your most treasured gift—as the apple of your eye? God gives us worth and dignity in creating us in His image; we must pass this worth and dignity on to our children. It will begin with our children observing our life and following our actions; it must lead to an understanding that you, as the parent, are attempting to mirror the lifestyle of Jesus Christ; it will hopefully end with a child's decision to follow Christ directly as their ultimate example.

Parents, we are mediators! Similar to Jesus showing us the way to the Father, we are to show our children the way to Jesus. The time will come soon enough when they will be mature enough to follow Christ directly. It is every Christian parent's utmost desire to see this transformation take place. As John the Baptist states in the Gospel of John 3:30, "He [Jesus Christ] must become greater; I [John the Baptist] must become less."

Paul, while writing to the young believers in Corinth, states in 1 Corinthians 4:14–16 (emphasis added), "I am not writing this to shame you, but to warn you, as my dear children. Even though you have ten thousand guardians in Christ, you do not have many fathers, for in Christ Jesus I became your father through the gospel. Therefore I urge you to *imitate* me." The apostle Paul was not afraid to take the lead and model his life as an example for these young believers. Parents, neither should we! Are you willing to say to your children, *"Follow me as I follow Christ"*?

When this transformation takes place, our responsibility is not over; instead, our role simply changes from being the direct example of the one each child is to emulate to a secondary role of encouragement and support. Both roles are necessary and are equally important.

Guess what? Our life song will still matter. We will always be an example to our children. So remember these three things: (1) It is never too early to be an example of Jesus to your children. (2) As your children mature and grow, help them develop a personal relationship with Jesus and encourage them to use Him as their ultimate example. (3) Teach your children that they are created in God's image and that He wants them to become transformed into God's likeness, going from drinking infant milk to eating solid food (Heb. 5:12-14)—to realize their worth and dignity to God.

I will end this section with the words from my favorite song, "My Buddy." The words are recorded with permission from Scott Springer, writer and lead singer of the Christian music group Halo.

> Pointing in endless directions, looking lost as a pup
> Reaching out for my hand, falling, then getting up
> Tugging on my trousers, crying for his way
> My little boy is growing; he looked like me today
> He looked like me today

My buddy sees me living; my buddy sees me fall
My buddy is a mirror, hanging on the wall
My buddy sees me silent; my buddy hears me talk
And my buddy will see Jesus, if in His life I walk

Mocking all my motions, he learns how to live
Walking in my footsteps, hearing advice I give
Sometimes I sit and wonder, just where with him I stand
A tear comes as I realize, his life is in my hands
His life is in my hands

My buddy sees me living; my buddy sees me fall
My buddy is a mirror, hanging on the wall
My buddy sees me silent; my buddy hears me talk
And my buddy will see Jesus, if in His life I walk

Now he's growing older, as he kneels to pray
He says, "God bless all your children,"
and then I hear him say,
He says, "Jesus, I love you, and for your love I'm glad
But there's just one thing I want to be, is just like my dad"

My buddy sees me living; my buddy sees me fall
My buddy is a mirror, hanging on the wall
My buddy sees me silent; my buddy hears me talk
And my buddy will see Jesus, if in His life I walk

9

Discipline and Repentance

BEFORE I BECAME A FATHER, I thought children didn't understand the difference between right and wrong until age four or five. Was I ever wrong! Somewhere between their ninth and twelfth month, my children mastered the art of innocent disobedience—you know, the "Gee, Dad, my arm spastically moved and threw those yummy vegetables on the floor" move. This was often times followed by the "Give me a break, Dad, I'm too young to remember what you just told me not to do" look.

By the age of eighteen months, my sweet, innocent babies were looking me square in the eye and saying *no*! As Christian parents, we try various forms of discipline (communication, time-outs, spanking, removal of privileges, natural consequences, logical consequences, positive reinforcement) in an attempt to develop an authoritative (high support and high control) parenting style that we hope will effectively teach/train our children.

To complicate matters, God has granted our children *wonderful* and *unique* personalities that best learn from different forms of discipline. I believed I had this discipline thing down until I met my second child, who responds quite differently to my attempts at discipline than my first child. Then came my third child.

Jesus tells a wonderful parable about two brothers in Matthew 21:28–30. The father asked both sons to spend the day working in the vineyard. One son said, "I will," but never entered the vineyard; the other son said, "I will not," but spent the entire day working in the vineyard.

Do you have a child who tells you exactly what you want to hear (very respectful and kind) but struggles with honoring his/her commitment (lazy, forgetful, or too busy)?

Do you have a child who draws the battle line clear and loud (argumentative and loves to ask why) and yet his or her word is golden (very reliable and responsible)?

I have learned that some forms of discipline work well for one child but poorly for a different child. Does God discipline us all the same or differently? The answer is coming soon!

To make the discipline challenge even more exciting, our children are constantly maturing, which makes some forms obsolete (spanking) and other forms more effective (take away the car keys or cell phone). Does God's method of discipline with us change as we mature as Christians? Read the words of Jesus recorded in Luke 12:47–48 (emphasis added):

> That servant *who knows* his master's will and does not get ready or does not do what his master wants will be beaten with many blows. But the one *who does*

not know and does things deserving punishment will be beaten with few blows.
From everyone who has been given much,
much will be demanded; and from the
one who has been entrusted with much,
much more will be asked.

Our desire as parents should be to train our children to
know the master's will! As parents, we need to be careful that
"our will" is consistent with God's will so that our teaching
and training will be profitable. We need to use those discipline methods that most effectively cause godly sorrow
within our children and which most effectively encourage our children to avoid further negative behavior. These
methods will likely differ to some extent for each child, and
they will change as each child matures.

In the game of basketball, referees use a method called
the "accordion theory" to enforce discipline on the court.
The theory states that if you start the game with very firm
discipline (read many whistles) in the first quarter, you
establish control very early and are able to let the players
play (read fewer whistles) in the fourth quarter when the
game is on the line.

Basketball referees understand that to start a game
with very little discipline will lead to unacceptable behavior
in the fourth quarter (when the intensity and competitiveness of the game is at a peak). I believe parenting is very
similar. If we start with a firm line of discipline during the
early years, we can establish a clearly understood level of
acceptable behavior/play which will prepare our children

for acceptable behavior in their teenage years (when the intensity and competitiveness of life is at a peak).

Furthermore, we are able to reduce the need for restrictions and protection as each child demonstrates responsibility and self-control, so they may truly enjoy the fourth quarter of their life in our home. The start and the finish are key in every race and in every game and in disciplining our children.

So our goal in discipline becomes quite clear: as parents, we need to discipline—as God disciplines us—over issues that matter to God, in order to produce godly sorrow within our children resulting in changed behavior that is pleasing to the master (God). The goal of discipline is to make disciples!

> Endure hardship as discipline; God is treating you as sons. For what son is not disciplined by his father? If you are not disciplined (and everyone undergoes discipline), then you are illegitimate children and not true sons. Moreover, we have all had human fathers who disciplined us and we respected them for it. How much more should we submit to the Father of our spirits and live! Our fathers disciplined us for a little while as they thought best; but God disciplines us for our good, that we may share in His holiness. No discipline seems pleasant at the time, but painful. Later on, however, it produces a harvest

of righteousness and peace for those who
have been trained by it. (Heb. 12:7–11)

For discipline to be truly effective, it must contain three parameters. First, it must be *for the good of the child.* The purpose of discipline is not to induce physical pain; it is simply to communicate a wrong behavior. Many young children are very tenderhearted and will cry at a tap to their behind or to the top of their hand. The tears they shed should be caused by recognizing they have not followed their parents' will rather than from the physical pain of a spanking.

Please, never discipline out of anger toward your child, and never slap a child in the face. This will communicate aggression causing your child to fear, rather than communicate poor behavior causing your child to obey. God disciplines us in love!

Second, *love and acceptance must never be held back* during or after discipline. My children often ran into my arms, for a hug, after being disciplined because they needed to know they were still loved and cherished by me. This is a natural response for many children when discipline is administered properly.

Third, *discipline must be reflected as training.* Spring training, training camps, new hire training and basic training serve the same purpose—preparation for the battle/ work that counts. Those training us expect us to struggle and fail. Eyes need to be upon us; ears need to listen to us; words need to be spoken; correct actions need to be demonstrated; disposition/attitude needs to be modeled;

skills need to be practiced again and again; and, yes, discipline needs to be consistently applied. Why? So we can be successful in the battle/work.

As we demonstrate our confidence and competence, and as we prove to be responsible and reliable, restrictions are relaxed and we are trusted to positively contribute to our team, family and society. Spiritual warfare is very real and, as parents, we need to train and prepare our children for attacks from the enemy of their soul—who knows their weaknesses and hot buttons. The best way to do this is with patience and loving kindness!

My eight-year-old son would enter his room very upset with me after being sent there for a time of correction and reflection. I encouraged him to discuss his behavior with God while sitting on his bed and would give him an appropriate verse to look up while "he served his time." I helped him highlight six verses of appropriate conduct (these became life verses for him) and I helped him memorize these verses (Eph. 4:28, 29; Phil. 2:14; Col. 3:9; 1 Thess. 5:16-18; James 1:19; 1 John 4:11).

Nine times out of ten, Caleb would come downstairs and give me a hug and an apology for his poor conduct. Romans 2:4 tells us that it is God's kindness, and patience, that lead a sinner toward repentance. Discipline takes time. Discipline takes teaching. Discipline takes coaching and counseling. *Parents, we must take the time necessary to administer proper discipline for our children's benefit.*

The story of the Prodigal Son (Luke 15:11–32) is a perfect example of discipline for the good of the child and of love and acceptance for the child. The father planned the party and ran to greet his son before he knew of any changed behavior. His love was not conditional to a proper response.

Leave behind any anger; leave behind any manipulation. Simply choose to discipline as our Heavenly Father does—with *love* for the *good* of the child.

Parents need to do more than simply talk to their child. Saying ("Hey, Johnny, why did you kick little Bobby in the head? Please don't do that again. Next time you are angry, throw a ball against a wall.") is not enough. Some form of negative consequence must accompany our words. Talking about unacceptable behavior can certainly be helpful; however, I fear that some parents use this communication as a way of escaping the personal pain and time commitment associated with disciplining their children.

One day, my two-year-old daughter walked up to her six-year-old sister, Rebekah, (seated on the floor combing her hair) grabbed her hair and yanked with all her might. My six-year-old sat and cried. She was smart enough not to do this to her eight year-old brother, whose response would have been very different. My two-year-old ran because she knew her act of aggression was not acceptable. I did not sit her down and ask her to please refrain from such behavior in the future—she knew what she did was wrong (and hid, like Adam and Eve in the garden).

Instead, I invested the time necessary to discipline her (a well-deserved time-out). Before I could utter any words, after her time-out, Sarah went immediately to her sister, gave her multiple kisses on her head, rubbed her head, and told her she was sorry.

Discipline measures, such as controlled spanking, time-outs, and ignoring unacceptable behavior (like temper tantrums), are not barbaric when administered in love, with the intent being one of communication rather than hurt, to the child. Proper discipline is an act of love.

I do not consider myself an expert on the subject of disciplining children, and my experience—raising three children—hardly qualifies me for any award nominations; however, I can read the Bible and attempt to follow the pattern of my Heavenly Father. My conclusion: avoid the extremes! Never discipline for personal gain (soothe anger, force behavior); never discipline to mold a child into being like you or to learn to fear you (the Sound of Music syndrome); never avoid discipline because it is too hard or time consuming (lazy, indifferent).

Discipline because you love the child and you desire to communicate acceptable behavior. Proverbs 3:11–12 states, "My son, do not despise the LORD's discipline and do not resent His rebuke, because the LORD disciplines those He loves, as a father the son He delights in."

Romans 2:4b states that "God's kindness leads (us) toward repentance." Because of the character of his father, the prodigal son knew that he could return to his father— at least as a servant. To his delight, his father—representing God in this story—welcomed him home as his son with open arms.

Teamwork is critical in the discipline process for two-parent families. Parents should expect their young children to make hurtful statements to them (on occasion) and to play one parent against the other (often). This is a natural response and should be met with firm, loving, and direct communication. Parents must let their children know that discipline is not a game to win or lose, and that Mom and Dad and child are all on the same team.

When a child is upset at one parent, it is important for the other parent to not become the "excuse maker" or "silent friend." The *other* parent should encourage the child to express his/her (fill in the emotion or feeling here) directly with the parent they are upset with. Third party "negotiating" often leads to a pattern of behavior that may become the norm. This will lead to a poor "communication" relationship in the long run.

Keep in mind that, especially during the preteen years, children will often view each parent through the eyes of their other parent. This is why parents must refrain from name calling and negative remarks about/to one another in front of the children (avoiding them completely is the higher goal). This is not to say that parents can't disagree with one another in public—they need to show respect and friendship in the way they disagree. Our children learn much by watching the way parents interact with one another. Learning how to resolve conflict (in a kind and caring way) is a very important lesson each child needs to learn.

The apostle Paul recorded a wonderful passage on repentance in 2 Corinthians 7:8–11 (emphasis added). Some background will be helpful. False teachers in Corinth were challenging Paul's personal integrity and his authority as an apostle. Many of the flock were falling astray to these false teachers. Paul writes the Corinthian believers a letter with the purpose being to change their behavior.

Even if I caused you sorrow by my letter, I do not regret it. Though I did regret it—I see that my letter hurt you, but only for a little while—yet now I am happy, not because you were made sorry, but because your sorrow led you to repentance. For you became sorrowful as God intended and so were not harmed in any way by us. *Godly sorrow brings repentance that leads to salvation and leaves no regret,* but worldly sorrow brings death. See what this *godly sorrow* has produced in you: what earnestness, what eagerness to clear yourselves, what indignation, what alarm, what longing, what concern, what readiness to see justice done. At every point you have proved yourselves to be innocent in this matter."

Was this letter easy for Paul to write? Wouldn't it have been much easier to ignore this behavior and hope that it would change with time? Read what Paul says about this letter in 2 Corinthians 2:4, "For I wrote you out of great distress and anguish of heart and with many tears, not to grieve you but to let you know the depth of my love for you."

Discipline is never easy to give or receive; however, kindness and good communication lead toward repentance. Repentance must always be accompanied by forgiveness. This basic Gospel message must penetrate every fiber of our being, every action we commit, every thought we possess.

Parents, the next time you become frustrated or angry at the actions of your child, ask yourself two questions. *Question 1*: Why are you frustrated/angry/hurt? *Question 2*: Does our Heavenly Father feel the same whenever we do wrong? Sometimes the action is performed out of ignorance (touching a hot stove); sometimes the action is performed out of defiance (battle of the wills).

How does our Heavenly Father feel when we sin because we don't understand why the Bible says we should not do something or why we should do something? How does our Heavenly Father feel when we sin because we desire to sin and care less about hurting God?

I see a remarkable parallel between my children's acts of disobedience (ignorance or defiance) and my own. I am truly challenged by my Heavenly Father's patience, kindness, and tolerance toward me in His discipline. Does God feel hurt when I disobey? Does God feel joy when I repent? The father of the prodigal sure did!

Should our response to discipline and repentance be like the slave who had millions of dollars of debt canceled, only to throw a friend in jail for a debt of several dollars hours later? No! Our response should be like King David in Psalm 51:1–4:

> Have mercy on me, O God, according to your unfailing love; according to your great compassion blot out my transgressions. Wash away all my iniquity and cleanse me from my sin. For I know my transgressions, and my sin is always before

me. Against you, you only, have I sinned
and done what is evil in your sight, so that
you are proved right when you speak and
justified when you judge.

God's discipline, and the hopeful response of our children to our discipline, can be summarized in one simple yet powerful word: *humility*.

Matthew 18: 1–4 says it best:

At that time the disciples came to Jesus and asked, "who is the greatest in the kingdom of heaven?" He called a little child and had him stand among them. And he said: "I tell you the truth, unless you change and become like little children, you will never enter the kingdom of heaven. Therefore, whoever *humbles* himself like this child is the greatest in the kingdom of heaven." (emphasis added)

Parents, we can learn much from our children!

I would like to share some personal long-term thoughts on parenting children as they move from adolescence to young adulthood through to adulthood. I try to involve my children in the decision-making process for their problems (as parents we need to resist the temptation of taking ownership for their problems) as soon as they are able to participate. For example, if they miss an assignment, I do not make excuses for them to their teacher or do their homework for them—I ask them how *they* plan on fixing *their* problem. I then limit my response to one of the following three (assuming they actually try to solve the problem and not say "I don't know"):

(A) This is a decision I agree with and will fully support.
(B) This is a decision that has risk and reward attached to it. I help them understand the risk and the reward—and the likelihood of either or both— and tell them I will support whatever they decide to do. *Side note*: We need not fear allowing our children to try and fail when the consequences are still minor. Better they learn this lesson at the earliest age possible.

I took Caleb to a baseball game when he was ten years old, and he had the opportunity to go to a short line and try for Richie Sexson's autograph (good player) or to the very long line and hope to get Tony Gwynn's autograph (Hall of Famer). We discussed the risk and reward, and he chose to go for Tony Gwynn's autograph. I figured he would return with no autograph and I could use that as a teachable moment. Predictably, Caleb never reached the dugout for Tony to sign before the National Anthem started and everyone returned to their seats. Everyone that is, except for Caleb. He moved to the top of the dugout and awaited Tony Gwynn to return (a highly unlikely outcome). He got Tony Gwynn's autograph and the ball sits proudly on display in his room still today. I took the opportunity to praise him for having a dream and going for it.

(C) This is a decision I cannot support (and give reason attached to it, such as morally wrong, too much financial or relational risk for too little reward, long-term disaster waiting to happen, etc.).

I think this format can continue as the kids move out of the house. I believe the key is being able to disagree without becoming disagreeable. *Not supporting a poor decision does not equate with not supporting my child*—although they could see it that way for a period of time.

I want to take a moment to talk about punishment versus discipline. In Scripture, punishment is linked to "hell," "the sword," "fire," "evil," "iniquity," and "disobedience." First John 4:18 (emphasis added) states, "There is no fear in love; but perfect love casts out fear, because fear involves *punishment*, and the one who fears is not perfected in love."

Hebrews 12:6 (emphasis added) tells us that "God *disciplines* those he loves." First Corinthians 11:32 (emphasis added) says, "But when we are judged, we are *disciplined* by the Lord in order that we may not be condemned (*punished*) along with the world." Proverbs instructs parents to *discipline* their children and for children to not resist the *discipline* of the Lord.

Near as I can tell, parents are encouraged to discipline their children, not punish their children. I think punishment is linked to the judicial system—God as Judge will punish the world (unbelievers). God as Judge will punish Satan and the fallen angels. Our US judicial system punishes wrongdoers with prison or even death for crimes against society.

As parents, we need to recognize that our children belong to God so we are called to discipline, to teach, and to train our children to stay away from eternal or societal punishment. God and societal judicial systems have the ultimate responsibility and right to exert punishment. I believe effective parenting/teaching focuses upon discipline. Discipline requires more time and effort on the part of the parent and leads to repentance and forgiveness. Punishment, on the other hand, usually leads to feelings of guilt and shame.

When I think of discipline, I think of 1 Timothy 3:16–17: "All Scripture is inspired by God and profitable for teaching, for reproof, for correction, for training in righteousness—that the man of God may be adequate, equipped for every good work" (let's not miss verse 17—the purpose for it). Discipline has all these components—teaching, reproof, correction, and training—to equip us!

God's discipline, and the hopeful response of our children to our discipline, can be summarized in one simple yet powerful word: *humility*.

10

One Another

"One Another" is two words in English, but it is only one word in Greek. It is used one hundred times in the New Testament. The usual context is one of love, unity and humility. Romans 12:10 states: "Be devoted to *one another* in brotherly love. Honor *one another* above yourselves" (emphasis added).

My wonderful children taught me the meaning of "one another". As a single man, I was typically selfish and focused on my own desires (usually watching and playing sports). I got married and started to learn how to share my time, my passions and my life with my wife, Regina. I had children and truly began to learn about being devoted to my family.

I made sacrifices as any good father does, and I have zero regrets. My children kept building a family dynamic built upon love and unity that made me yearn to be a better man. The dedication, care and loyalty they have for one another is truly inspiring.

Each child is uniquely gifted with talents, personalities and leadership qualities; yet, they fit perfectly together as a team – better yet, a family! They each had special names we gave them to match their amusing temperaments. Caleb (C-Dawg) is our loyal lab who looks out for his sisters and enjoys being with them (he attends all their events, cheering them on wildly); Rebekah (our Otter daughter) loves to play and is constantly singing, dancing and laughing; and Sarah (Raccoon) who has off the chart street smarts, knows how to get into and out of challenges better than anyone I know. She is also the best athlete in our family.

These three siblings formed a bond of trust with one another to the point we could not get them to tattle (I did not find out who broke the window until I was over 50 years old). When times were good, they shared with each other, then mom and dad. When times were tough, they shared with each other, and sometimes mom and dad. During sharing time at meals, they truly cared about one another's day.

One of my favorite memories happened in elementary school when Caleb was in sixth grade and Rebekah was in fourth grade. The school bully was mean to Rebekah and called her a name, making her cry. She ran to her brother. Caleb told the bully to apologize to his sister. The bully pushed Caleb to the pavement, skinning his knee and elbow. Caleb was an instant hero to Rebekah. The next day the bully approached Caleb and told him he respected him for standing up for his sister and never bothered either of them again. Here is my favorite part: when Sarah was in elementary school several years later, and a bully threatened her, she came home and shared her story with us over dinner. I offered to intervene and Sarah told me she would rather have Caleb come to her school because the bully might hurt me.

To this very day, with my children grown and out of the home, my children continue to support, share with and comfort one another – still often before calling mom and dad. They even have special handshakes when they greet each other. I would have it no other way! As siblings, they share a special bond that parents need to promote and nurture.

With regard to "one another", the Bible tells us to be devoted to, honor, love, have fellowship with, live in peace with, be gentle with, encourage and build-up, comfort, bear burdens, forgive, accept, bear with, be kind to, submit to, speak truthfully with, offer hospitality to, teach and admonish, serve and pray for. Look at these commands. Can you imagine a home full of family members who are dedicated to doing this with and for one another?

My children taught me in their prayers that it is okay to tell God everything and anything and to do so every night, as well as being sure to pray for each family member by name; they taught me about devotion as they gave a gift to Jesus each Christmas (song, poem, acts of service) before ever opening any presents themselves—in fact, they would spend their AWANA bucks buying presents for each other and graduated to real money as they got older (the gift from a sibling carried extra significance); they gathered together for hours each Christmas morning in one of their rooms, before coming to see mom and dad; they taught me how to serve by attending international mission trips together and ultimately attending Biola University together; and they taught me how to love one another as they truly cared for and supported each other.

My children taught me what it means to be an advocate. Job 16:19-21 states: "Even now my witness is in heaven; my advocate is on high. *My intercessor is my friend* as my eyes pour out tears to God; on behalf of a man he pleads with God as a man pleads for his friend" (emphasis mine). When one of my children was being disciplined with a time-out or a logical consequence restriction, they did not come to mom or dad and beg for mercy—their sibling did this for them. They reminded me of the good they have done, the sorrow they feel and that they belong to our family. Hebrews Chapter 7 describes Jesus interceding for us in a similar way with the Father—Jesus says they belong to me!

My children taught me how to bear with and forgive one another. Obviously, none of them are perfect and each had their moments pushing buttons and getting their buttons pushed. But, their devotion and love for one another caused them to choose the relationship over the principle and to solve the conflict, rather than avoid or exacerbate it. My wife and I paid attention, listened and learned. We did not believe in playing the role of referee or counselor. When conflict was evident, we sent them to a room together and told them to figure it out and to not leave the room until they did so. My two oldest children became Communication majors. My youngest is studying to become a licensed Marriage and Family Therapist. Learning conflict resolution skills at a young age is very important. Here is a nugget of truth: they begin learning by watching mom and dad.

Did you ever stop to ponder that our children are blessed with siblings to help them develop Emotional Intelligence? The five pillars of Emotional Intelligence are: Self-Awareness (knows own strengths/weaknesses/needs/drives/moods and hot buttons); Self-Regulation (control of feelings; trustworthy; integrity; thinks before taking action); Motivation (driven to achieve; passionate; persistent; optimistic; unconditional commitment to the team); Empathy (thoughtful; considerate; appreciative of uniqueness; gives individualized attention; sensitive to needs of others); and Social Skill (good communicator; persuasive; friendliness with a purpose; builds relationship with rapport).

These attributes require "one another" to help us nurture and develop them into our lives. Once we discover our sibling, we begin to realize that the world truly does not revolve just around us. We begin learning how to manage our self and our feelings, and how to care about others and their feelings. Our motivation becomes less self-driven and hopefully, more team (or family) driven – "Holden" becomes more prominent and important than "Dave"!

We start developing empathy by learning how to become considerate, thoughtful and sensitive to the feelings of our siblings. We learn how to engage in active listening and the importance of sharing and caring. These life skills help us become successful in school, at work, in marriage and in any mission field. These life skills are universally recognized as top qualities of great leadership.

It all starts with our relationship with our siblings (or other children our age) and it continues with team sports, school, youth groups, and other team-oriented organizations. It requires parenting with a purpose: choosing to teach and train our children in the way they should go (Proverbs 22:6); choosing to spend dedicated time building character qualities, like emotional intelligence, into each child's life (Proverbs 20:11); and choosing to cultivate the family relationships God has blessed you with, to nurture sibling connections, by developing honor and promoting teamwork (Proverbs 17:17).

My children taught me that the Christian life is not to be lived in isolation; rather, it is to be lived in inclusion with one another.

We start developing empathy by learning how to become considerate, thoughtful and sensitive to the feelings of our siblings.

11

Time

IT IS IMPOSSIBLE TO SEPARATE our *time* commitments from our order of priority. Break down 720 hours (thirty days times twenty-four hours per day) for a given month and allocate it into categories of how you use it. A great feature of time is that it is consistent and impartial. Everybody has an equal allotment; we choose how to *use* it.

A horrible feature of time is that it is consistent and impartial. Everybody has an equal allotment; we choose how to *abuse* it. The people with too much time (bored) can't give it away, and the people with not enough time (burnt) can't purchase any extra.

Unfortunately for many, by the time we realize that our priorities are out of whack, our children are grown and no longer want/need our time. Our busy schedule has left us with a damaged marriage, disillusioned with the corporate ladder of success, and unable to communicate with our children.

Our children especially require our time during their preteen years. Think of each child as a young oak tree. They require sunlight, water, and a fertile ground with deep soil.

The sunlight represents the spiritual and emotional nutrients. The water represents the physical and mental nutrients. The deep soil represents the opportunity to grow.

The early years are critical for the oak tree to establish firm, healthy, deep roots so extensive growth may occur later. An oak tree afforded good sunlight and water will still die without good soil. We, as parents, are responsible to provide each child with good, deep soil (read secure, loving environment) so the roots may grow strong and deep enough to weather future storms they will encounter in life.

The early years of growth for a strong and healthy oak tree require more time and maintenance than the latter years; hence, lack of time spent cultivating the soil will produce a sick oak tree in need of much maintenance in the latter years.

Parents, spend the time now while your young oak tree is still establishing its roots. Isaiah 61:3 gives us a glimpse of God's plan for His children: "They will be called oaks of righteousness, a planting of the LORD for the display of His splendor."

We may ask ourselves, *why did we have children?* If the answer is to raise and enjoy them, then why don't/didn't we? Do not blame other people or other things for *your* failure to control *your* time. Let me soften that statement: *Please* do not blame other people or other things for *your* failure to control *your* time. This statement applies to myself as much as anyone else; I don't like to face the fact that how I spend my time is my choice either.

Did God make a mistake in giving us only twenty-four hours each day? I don't believe so. I would just as easily fill-up a thirty-hour day and complain about having no time. Before I sound too harsh, I must recognize that events will come into our lives that will turn any schedule upside down. We will all battle storms in this life. I am talking about the day in/day out grind of life that is within our control.

Below I will evaluate six "time mongers" that we all face in our everyday life. There exists many "time fillers," such as television, reading, social media, various hobbies, etc.; however, the six "time mongers" are without question all good, healthy things that we should be involved with. The question is how to balance and prioritize rather than what to limit or eliminate.

Life necessities—eating, drinking, sleeping, and hygiene. We all must spend daily time in these areas for mere survival. Jesus certainly, with the exception of periods of fasting, spent daily time on these necessities of life. This area is usually not a problem until we abuse other areas and soon pay the consequences. When our eating and sleeping patterns become inconsistent because we need to "save some time," our health begins to fail and we lose more time (sluggish, lethargic, famished, weak) than we ended up saving.

Other people and other projects suffer from our lack of sharpness/energy as well. How many times in the Bible do we read about Jesus being unable to function due to malnourishment or fatigue? I can think of two—after forty days of fasting and temptation in the desert and after being flogged and encountering multiple beatings on the road to Calvary. Other than those two storms—signifying the beginning and the end of His earthly ministry, the Bible shows Him to be a man of incredible energy and strength. The message is simple—trying to cut corners and save time by skipping meals and sleep for a prolonged period of time will only lead to deteriorated health and more time needed for recovery.

Work and/or school are also necessities that we are able to control our spent time. How, you may ask? Most jobs require forty to fifty hours per week. This is manageable! Extra hours spent above and beyond this time commitment need to be heavily weighed. What is your ROI (return on investment)? Does the extra money or the extra prestige or the extra enjoyment outweigh the sacrifices you make in your time?

In other words, does the opportunity cost of what else you could be doing with your time warrant those extra hours you spend at work or in school? If those hours must be spent in order to allow your spouse to stay at home with your children, you are building with gold, silver, and costly stones. If, however, those extra hours are spent chasing honors, possessions, compliments, or titles, you are building with wood, hay, and straw (1 Cor. 3:12), leaving you with a very weak ROI!

Consider these possibilities. Taking fewer units and graduating later. Turning down a job promotion that offers more discretionary income but requires more of your time. Learning how to delegate and train. Asking your wife and children if the ROI is worth the time commitment. Keep in mind that our work and school relationships are temporal; our relationship with our wife and children are eternal for those who know the LORD.

Friends and social activities—scheduled and unscheduled, they take up time. This is not bad. Jesus spent time with friends (Lazarus, Mary, and Martha) and attended social gatherings (weddings, dinner parties). How involved are your spouse and children in these events? Are they included or does this take time away from them? I am not advocating zero friendships and zero social gatherings; I am advocating the need for moderation and prioritizing. The desire to raise and enjoy children requires this.

Exercise is healthy for the body and the mind. All too often exercise is placed before our family. It happens so quickly and easily that we hardly recognize it. We join a gym and attend three nights a week, we play one night a week on the church softball team, and we play basketball Saturday morning with the guys at the local Bible college gym. We then tell our children that we don't have time to play with them because we have to bring home the bacon for our family to live on. I struggled with this one.

Exercise is a great stress release and helps keep us mentally sharp and alert and in good shape physically. The question is, how much is enough? You must answer that yourself! Opportunity cost? ROI? Consider this: coaching your child's sports team or exercising together as a family (tennis, bicycle riding, walking). What profits the man or woman who gains an in-shape body yet forfeits time spent with his family? I certainly understand the desire to "play with the guys/gals"—just don't go overboard and forsake your family.

Church fellowship and involvement—a must for the spiritually mature. God has equipped and gifted every one of us to serve in His kingdom. Can we overcommit to service and church fellowship? Yes, we can! If you are continually telling your family that you do not have time for them because you are busy serving God, you are missing the boat—better yet, you have missed the entire dock! Your first service to God as a spouse and parent is to provide for and love your family.

Let's look at Jesus as our example again. He committed Himself to twelve men—we commonly refer to them as the twelve disciples. This was Jesus' family. Did Jesus spend all His time performing miracles, evangelizing the lost, and healing the sick and lame? *No!* He spent much of His time training these disciples to carry on His Father's work after He left this world. Are we training our children to carry on the work of our Father? This requires *time!*

Listen to the words of Jesus as He prays for His disciples recorded in John 17:6–12 (emphasis added):

> I have revealed you to those whom you gave me out of the world. They were yours; you gave them to me and they have obeyed your work. Now they know that everything you have given me comes from you. For I gave them the words you gave me and they accepted them. They knew with certainty that I came from you, and they believed that you sent me. I pray for them. *I am not praying for the world, but for*

those you have given me, for they are yours. All I have is yours, and all you have is mine. And glory has come to me through them. I will remain in the world no longer, but they are still in the world, and I am coming to you. Holy Father, protect them by the power of your name—the name you gave me—so that they may be one as we are one. While I was with them, I protected them and kept them safe by that name you gave me. None has been lost except the one doomed to destruction so that Scripture would be fulfilled.

What an awesome way to view our family: gifts from God that belong to Him but are placed under our care. This viewpoint denotes both worth and responsibility for our family. Our response must become one of humility and obedience. It is not a matter of success or failure, it is simply a willingness to raise and enjoy this gift.

Worship/devotions/personal growth—a must to obtain and maintain spiritual maturity. I am definitely guilty of cutting corners in this area to save time for the other areas. The result: I find myself less patient, less joyful, less able to cope with stress and feeling guilty about my lack of quality prayer time. This area was so easy for me as a single college student; it became a challenge to manage after marriage; it has become all too inconsistent after children.

My words of wisdom and insight in this area are simple and few: this area is holy and sacred and must be maintained. Do not sacrifice this area to gain more time. "Immediately Jesus made the disciples get into the boat and go on ahead of Him to the other side, while He dismissed the crowd. After He had dismissed them, He went up on a mountainside by Himself to pray…" (Matt. 14:22–23).

I know these "time mongers" all too well. I blinked and I was missing milestone moments because I was too busy. So I decided to self-prune my schedule. I turned down job opportunities and promotions; I took fewer units in school each semester on my 2nd degree and delayed working on my Masters until my children were all in their teens; I stopped playing on my travel church softball team and started Coaching my children instead; I included my children in exercising; I accepted the Church leadership positions that included family; and I began hanging out with other young families where children were always welcome.

I did make some personal sacrifices; however, the gains of spending the extra time with my family – instead of away from my family – was a much bigger ROI, leading to a greater feeling of fulfillment and joy. I have no regrets! As my children matured thru their high school and college years: I went back and got my Masters, I rejoined my Church softball team, I went back to the gym three nights a week, I accepted more leadership opportunities with my church and I began double-dating with other empty nest couples. You see, the opportunities never went away for me. My priorities simply changed. I thank my children for teaching me how to prioritize my time – with them!

Time is an earthly trust, which, if invested wisely, will produce eternal treasures. Time is a limited resource extended only by giving the first part back to God. Time is a daily treasure that attracts many robbers. Our Heavenly Father has equipped us with gifts; He has given us the assignment of extending His kingdom; and He has given us time to fulfill this mission. The best place to start is with our family.

What an awesome way to view our family: gifts from God that belong to Him but are placed under our care.

12

Stewardship

WHY DID GOD CREATE MANKIND? Was He lonely? Was He bored? Or did He simply have the desire for a new relationship? I have often wondered why God waited six days into creation to fulfill His objective of making mankind. I think I finally understand. Before there can be a *people*, there must be a *place*. So God spent five days creating the heavens and the earth for us. How cool!

And while mankind continues to argue the point and origin of its existence, the Bible clearly teaches us that our time here on earth is temporary: "Just as man is destined to die once, and after that to face judgment" (Heb. 9:27). The Bible also clearly teaches us that we are created by God: "The LORD God formed the man from the dust of the ground and breathed into his nostrils the breath of life, and man became a living being" (Gen. 2:7).

The Bible further explains that God created man in His own image (Gen. 1:27) and God created woman so man would not be alone (Gen. 2:18). So what does all this mean? God is into relationships! The undeniable truth is God loves! He loves us and desires to be with us. He was not ordered to make us by some Cosmic Boss. He was not bored and in need of a new challenge. He didn't need slaves or servants, so He gave us free will. He simply desires and values relationships so deeply that He created a universe for us, and then He created us.

But God did even more than that. He created a training and learning ground, we call Earth, where we can learn how to love and how to be loved. God came down to Earth (Jesus) and lived with us for thirty-three and a half years providing mankind with the ultimate example of a loving relationship (John 3:16, 13:15, 15:9–13, 17:22–26). The plan is very simple: (1) Begin life as an infant and learn about God's love. (2) Grow and learn how to demonstrate this love toward others. (3) Share God's love with people who do not know God personally.

The flow chart goes something like this: Develop a relationship with God → Develop relationships with other people → Share your story.

I have often wondered why God gave mankind this training ground on Earth instead of starting us off in heaven with Him. I believe it is because a major requirement for a love relationship to develop is "freedom of choice." In order for mankind to learn how to love and how to be loved, opposite choices such as hatred, rejection, and fear must be present. These opposite choices cannot dwell in heaven with God (study the removal of Lucifer and one-third of the angels). In order for love to be *real*, it must be *free*!

The spiritual term for this training ground is *stewardship*. Stewardship is the management of God's resources. It is the proper understanding and recognition that God owns everything and we are His representatives or ambassadors. Second Corinthians 5:20 states, "We are therefore, Christ's ambassadors, as though God were making His appeal through us."

Our job here on earth is to manage the resources God gives to us (see Gen. 2:15 and Matt. 21:33–44). I believe this includes the children He blesses us with. Although we refer to them as our children, they truly belong to God first! Again, the perfect example is that of Jesus. God gave Jesus human parents (Joseph and Mary) to care for and nurture and teach Him; however, God is the ultimate authority/parent.

The same is true for our children. God is using us as stewards to care for and nurture and teach His children about His love and plans for their lives. I believe that when we keep this proper perspective, the priority we place upon raising our children, the love in which we discipline our children and the time we commit to spending with our children becomes more defined and something we enjoy.

God validates us as parents with great worth by entrusting us with His precious children. Jesus loves the little children, all the children of the world—red, brown, yellow, black, and white, they are precious in his sight; Jesus loves the little children of the world.

Remember at the beginning of this chapter when I noted that before there can be a *people*, there must first be a *place*? Read the incredible words of Jesus recorded in John 14:1–3 (emphasis added).

"Do not let your hearts be troubled. Trust in God; trust also in me. In my Father's house are many rooms; if it were not so, I would have told you. I am going there to *prepare a place* for you. And if I go and *prepare a place* for you, I will come back and take you to be with me that you also may be where I am."

God's plan is for mankind to learn how to develop "real love" relationships, to choose them freely, and to enjoy them for eternity. So how does this plan apply to you as a parent?

Your Heavenly Father has fashioned by hand for you children to enjoy and teach. These are the primary responsibilities for you as a parent. Are you enjoying your children as they grow up? Each year brings a new challenge and a new depth to the relationship. Are you actively teaching your children about their past (how God created them), their present (how God wants to be with them every day), and their future (how God is preparing a place for them for eternity)? We have no guarantee how many hours, days, or years we will live together under the same roof at home—so start enjoying and teaching now while you have the opportunity to do so!

If you consider a child leaving home for college, at age eighteen, to be a realistic possibility for your child, as I did for mine, we are facing a reality that our child, upon reaching first grade, has lived one-third of his/her expected "life at home," and upon reaching fourth grade, this same child has lived one-half of his/her expected "life at home."

I love my children and enjoyed living with them so much that the thought of them leaving my home some day was overwhelming. But then I remember: in order for love to be *real*, it must first be *free*! My hope and desire is to build such a strong relationship with my children "today" that when God calls them away to begin their own families and/or vocation "tomorrow" they will still enjoy visiting home.

I am greatly saddened by how many Christian parents I know, who were raised in a Christian home, who have very little desire to visit with (or feel great stress from disapproval or unfulfilled expectations while visiting with) their parents.

I want my children excited to see me when they are grown and away. My relationship with them "tomorrow" will largely be determined by my relationship with them "today." I know that while time and schedules in this world today bind me, I cannot spend enough time with my children; my prayer is that they feel the same way about me.

I am a realist! I understood that during my child's teenage years, he/she would exercise more freedom and the quantity of our time together would decrease; however, the quality was still there and the love and enjoyment was real. For now, enjoy all the quantity you can with your young children while you are still cool!

For continued studies on this topic consider the following parent–child relationships recorded in the Bible.

<u>For Mothers:</u>
Mary and Jesus (unconditional love)
Moses and his mother (protection from evil)
Naomi and Ruth (relationship/commitment)
Timothy and Eunice (teaching/education)

<u>For Fathers:</u>
Abraham and Isaac (trust/obedience)
Jacob and Joseph (confidence/family heritage)
Prodigal son and his father (love/forgiveness)
Joseph and Jesus (skill/vocation)

God is using us as stewards to care for and nurture and teach His children about His love and plans for their lives.

13

Learning in Joy

YOUR FIRST DAY AT AN amusement park. Your first game of the season. Seeing the ocean for the first time. Jumping in the pool after four long months of winter. That new movie you have been waiting to see. The new CD released by your favorite group. The championship game. Exciting expectations breed joy!

Children seem particularly adept at enjoying the experience and at finding joy in the journey. Caleb played every game as though it were his first and his last. His competitive drive and pure enjoyment of playing combined to produce a joy that remained throughout the entire game. Rebekah would ride the roller coasters and laugh as long as the park remained open. Sarah just wanted to be involved and treated as part of the team. "Get a movie I can watch," "Play a game I can play," and "Let me stay up late with everyone" were some of her favorite statements.

Whether the experience is new or familiar, if it is fun and exciting, joy will follow. I believe that there is joy in learning *and* learning in joy! Parents are pretty good at enjoying the firsts of life and at discovering joy in learning, but children can teach parents much about discovering learning in joy. The Bible speaks of making our joy *complete* in at least five books (Deut. 16:15; John 15:11; Phil. 2:2; 1 John 1:4; 2 John 12).

I honestly believe that God intends for believers to sustain joy and to express joy on a daily basis. Why else would joy be a section of the fruit of the Spirit? Joy leads to praise. Look at Luke 10:21: "At that time Jesus, full of joy through the Holy Spirit, said, I praise you, Father…" As Christian parents, we should be full of joy and praise!

Do bad things happen? Do trials come? Is pain and hurt real? Do some days suck? The obvious answer is *yes*! But there is learning in joy. As we choose to focus upon what we do have rather than upon what we do not have; as we focus upon our eternal rewards rather than upon our temporary defeats. As we choose joy over despair, betterness over bitterness, and encouragement over discouragement, peace and contentment begin to encompass our being. And our joy becomes complete. And we learn.

I want to be sure I draw the distinction between joy and happiness. Happiness is a temporary emotion that naturally comes and goes with life's ups and downs. I was a very unhappy parent on several occasions (arguing, disobedience, lack of sleep, lack of appreciation, the list can go on); however, I could still choose to be joyful—recognizing that I would rather be a parent with some unhappy moments than not be a parent at all.

Despite displeasing God with my selfish behavior, my willful disobedience and my ungrateful heart attitude, I understand and know that my Heavenly Father never regretted creating me—in fact, He reminds me that I am fearfully and wonderfully made (Psalm 139:14). In John 16:21, Jesus states: "A woman giving birth to a child has pain because her time has come; but when her baby is born she forgets the anguish because of her *joy* that a child is born into the world" (emphasis mine).

A woman giving birth is not happy—trust me, I have been there; however, mom remains joyful because she has the long-term perspective of wisdom and understanding. Moms and dads who understand that parenting is a journey, rather than a destination, benefit greatly by allowing joy to become their strength.

In John Chapter 17, the words of Jesus praying to His Heavenly Father on the night of His arrest are recorded. In verse 13 He states: "I am coming to you now, but I say these things while I am still in the world, so that they may have the full measure of my *joy* within them" (emphasis mine). Do you see it? Jesus was about to be betrayed, tortured and killed—and he is still full of joy (because He knew what His death was about to accomplish).

And Jesus is asking for the full measure of joy to remain in His disciples who were about to experience the greatest grief and doubt in their lives. And His joy is complete even knowing His disciples are about to abandon, and in the case of Peter, deny Him.

As parents, we learn to forgive ourselves and to forgive one another for the mistakes we make rearing our children. We learn how to find strength to persevere during those late nights and early mornings. We learn to cherish every moment, with each child, appreciating the unique gifts God has woven into them.

I have so much fun going on family activities and I learn so much. My children teach me how to overcome the stress in my life; how to laugh and play as I tear down the inhibitions in my life; how to make decisions as a team unified in purpose and mind.

One night I awoke at 3:30 a.m. to the sound of my seven-year-old son reading in the hall. As I opened my door, I found him reading out loud his Bible using the bathroom light we always leave on. He was so excited for his first basketball game the next morning that he could not sleep. So he got out of bed at 2:00 a.m., grabbed his Bible, and started reading. He is excited about learning how to read in school and how to play basketball in his church league. The learning leads to joy and the joy leads to learning.

Mom and Dad, do you remember how your eyes sparkled on your graduation day, on your wedding day, and on the day of the birth of each child? Now watch your children play and experience new things. Do you see the same sparkle? First Thessalonians 5:16 says, "Be joyful always." God commands us to be joyful because He knows that every time we choose joy as our response to life's pleasures and problems: we learn, we mature, and we persevere. And our joy becomes complete!

Part III

What the Future Holds

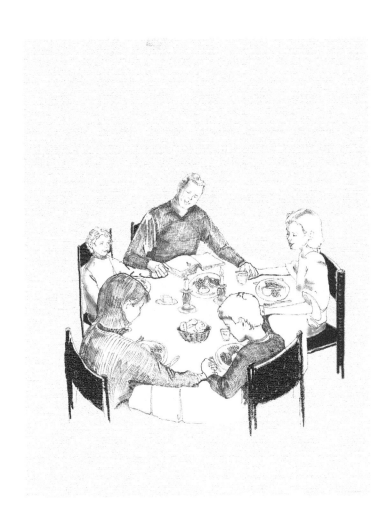

14

Purposeful Planning!

As CHRISTIANS, WE ARE TAUGHT early on our journey that God has a wonderful plan for our life. Jeremiah 29:11 states, "'For I know the plans I have for you,'" declares the Lord, "'plans to prosper you and not to harm you, plans to give you hope and a future.'"

As parents of elementary-aged children, we need to have a plan to give our children a hope and a future: a plan for their physical health (eating and exercise), a plan for their mental growth (education and endurance), a plan for their emotional needs (encouragement and empathy), and a plan for their spiritual welfare (evangelism, edification, and eternity).

F-15 Fighter pilots fly at more than seven hundred miles per hour just three hundred feet above the ground, tracking the enemy by radar, communicating with seven wingmen by radio, checking three hundred-plus cockpit instruments at nine G's while performing one mission. To be successful, the pilot must be prepared. The pilot starts with a *plan* (what are our objectives, threats, tactics?), moves to a *briefing* (how do we achieve our objectives, avoid our threats, and implement our tactics?), *executes* the plan as briefed (follows orders and prepares for contingencies), and has a *debriefing* (to analyze the execution, to calculate the cost, and to determine the effectiveness of the plan).

Mom and Dad, what is your plan for your child? What is God's plan for your child? Do these plans coincide? God had a purposeful plan for every person in the Bible (even for some of the animals). God used each parent to help prepare each child for His purpose. Take a look at the following model based loosely on the F-15 fighter pilot.

Plot

THE WORD *PLOT* DENOTES A greater purpose to be carried out in the future. We need to "plot out" the character traits, the skills, the know-how, the values that we want our child to possess by the time they leave our home (nest). How important is education, how important is work ethic, how important is physical training/athletic ability, how important is communication and relationship?

As parents, what are our mission objectives for each child? We desire servant leadership; we desire eternal dwelling with Jesus; we desire a Christian marriage with godly offspring; we desire good health, overflowing joy, and a fulfilling vocation.

What threats exist in this world to undermine our objectives? We have sinful nature, fiery darts from the evil one, and love of the world to overcome. What tactics do we possess? We have the Word of God, the indwelling of the

Holy Spirit, the Church, Christian resources, and hopefully godly grandparents.

One thing Regina and I greatly valued was a lasting, positive sibling relationship. It was very important to us that each child have an "excellent" relationship with his/her brother/sister today, tomorrow, and forever! We were very intentional in how we parented with this regard and made this a major plot in each child's life.

Inform

As PARENTS, WE NEED TO prepare, explain, instruct, and direct each child in the way he/she should go. Matthew 7:13–14 says, "Enter through the narrow gate. For wide is the gate and broad is the road that leads to destruction, and many enter through it. But small is the gate and narrow the road that leads to life, and only a few find it." We need to teach each child what we as parents value and what God values.

Our children need to be informed what is acceptable behavior and what is unacceptable behavior. Our children need to be informed what the consequences are for unacceptable behavior. This takes time. This takes purposeful planning. God has given us His word to instruct, Jesus as a model to follow, and the Holy Spirit to help us. As parents, we need to provide verbal and written instruction, be willing to model, and ready to help.

Regina and I very consistently taught our children the importance of having "excellent" sibling relationships with one another, we quickly dealt with any threats, and we used any and all tactics available to us to enforce this teaching.

Perform

AFTER WE DEVELOP THE PLOT and inform each child, we implement, execute, and complete the plan. This is where the rubber meets the road! We need to use checklists, establish mutual support for one another, and carry out the plot as informed.

We need to remain flexible as circumstances and outside forces change our landscape. We need to stay true to our original objective, yet be adaptable and prepared with contingencies. We need to inform our child of any change that comes and the new work-around to achieve our objective. For example, parents may plot to send their child to a private Christian college, but a financial disaster may make that plan impossible to achieve. What will you do? Did you have a contingency plan?

It is very important that parents remind one another of the objective (for example: need to save money today to help pay for college tuition tomorrow) and support one another during times of difficulty. Not every child agrees with every parent's plot. This is why it is very important the plot be consistent with scripture and adaptable to the unique gifts and desires God has placed within your child. Parents should never plot the vocation for their child; rather, they should encourage them to pursue honorable vocations that God has imprinted upon their heart and to become a servant leader who seeks to bring God glory.

Regina and I implemented several practices to keep our children in "excellent" relationship with one another. We had frequent family nights; our children attended one another's sporting, music, and drama events; we took family vacations together without bringing along friends; we talked in the car and did not permit iPods or iPhones when together; we ate together as a family; we prayed together as a family; we respected one another's person and property; we recognized our children when they encouraged one another without prompting.

Regina and I have had many parents comment to us on how well our children get along with one another and how nice it is to see brothers and sisters as best friends. This does not happen by accident. It is part of each child's plot.

Evaluate

ACCOUNTABILITY AND EXAMINATION ARE PART of any successful plot. Second Corinthians 13:5 says, "Examine yourselves to see whether you are in the faith; test yourselves…" We need frequent performance evaluations to see how well our objectives are being met. We need to be ready to measure, gauge, calculate, determine, and compute our plot. We need to be willing to reexamine our plot to see if it can be made more specific, more measurable, and more achievable.

We do this as employees at work with our projects. We do this as coaches on the court or ball field with our players. We need to do this as parents in the home with our child. We need to encourage the child to help develop the plot so they are more likely to perform the plot. We need to receive input from our child as we evaluate our plot. What lessons have we learned and how close are we to accomplishing each objective?

Regina and I scheduled "alone" time to discuss— to evaluate—our plot, our objectives for each child. Sometimes we went out to eat. Sometimes we left the kids with the grandparents and went away for a couple of nights. Sometimes we called each other on the cell phone or at work to quickly update each other. All these conversations were part of the evaluation process. Sometimes we only needed a minute, sometimes we needed an evening, and other times required a weekend away.

The key is consistent communication that is planned and purposeful.

15

Are There Any Guarantees?

"Train a child in the way he should go, and when he is old he will not turn from it" (Prov. 22:6). Is the verse recorded above an absolute promise for Christian parents? Can a solid biblical upbringing guarantee one's salvation? The answer to the above questions is *no!* The verse does not claim to be an absolute. Proverbs 22:6 must be understood within the context of free will. Ultimately, no person or system can guarantee the salvation for another. Only an active personal relationship with Jesus Christ can guarantee salvation. The verse above does reveal a solid tendency, I believe.

The Old Testament promises curses and blessings through third and fourth generations based upon parental obedience/disobedience. Again, these verses must be understood within the context of mankind's free will and the grace of God. Parental disobedience to the word of God does not guarantee a hopeless life of "being lost" for their children; in the same way, parental obedience to the word of God does not guarantee a life filled with hope and salvation for their children.

They do reveal an inclination. I believe that each generation has a more *clear* decision to make. As a multi-generational Christian, I grew up attending church, singing about Jesus and praying to God before I even knew that I needed a Savior. The choice for Jesus seemed obvious and simple to me. I saw that it worked in the lives of my parents and grandparents so why wouldn't it work in mine?

Eventually, the time came when my parents' faith truly became my own. Many children who grow up in a Christian environment, full of love and joy in the church (and in the home as well), choose Jesus as their Lord and Savior; however, we need only remember the prodigal son to realize that there are no guarantees. The prodigal son did return, but many never do.

Similarly, children reared by parents who embrace sex, drugs, and alcohol as gods in their family also often choose the same. Praise God that His grace is sufficient for all and that none are beyond His love and forgiveness. Too many end up lost, but some have discovered the saving love of Jesus.

College-educated parents often have college-educated children. College-uneducated parents often have college-uneducated children. Wealthy parents often have children who spend adulthood in affluence. Poor parents often have children who struggle financially. There are no guarantees! Still, tendencies do exist. Certain cycles require stronger effort to overcome or break.

Parents, I believe that the more solid your relationship is with Jesus, your spouse, and your children, the more difficult the decision becomes for your child to choose a different way or direction. All three relationships are pivotal. If a relationship with Jesus is real, it will encompass your entire life, and it will guide every relationship you have. Children pick up on hypocrisy very easily. Church attendance is not enough—Jesus must make a difference fifty-two weeks a year, seven days a week, twenty-four hours a day.

Are there any guarantees? *No!* But you can make a difficult decision easier. Be willing to take a stand. Join Joshua in proclaiming, "Choose for yourselves this day whom you will serve…But as for me and my household, we will serve the Lord" (Josh. 24:15).

Okay! I will give you *one* guarantee. I guarantee you that after your children are mature and have graduated from your home, as you ponder your parenting years, you will *never* regret spending too much time loving, enjoying, and rearing your children. The truth is that many parents will wish they had spent more time enjoying the journey and less time "stressing out" or being "too busy."

One of my favorite stories resides in Luke 10:38-42. Jesus is visiting friends and two sisters are with them (Martha & Mary). Martha is "distracted by all the preparations" while Mary "sat at the Lord's feet". When Martha asks Jesus to tell Mary to help her, He responds with: "Mary has chosen what is better." My simple translation is: Relationships trump Preparations! Parents: please do not become so distracted preparing your child's future that you fail to simply enjoy spending quality, fun time living in the now with them.

Rearing children is like a vacation. Combine the right mix of time, planning, and flexibility and you have a lasting memory that floods your heart and soul with warmth. Rush through the same vacation (trying to do it all), have poor planning (we needed reservations?), or ignore/fight the surprises life brings (that was not on our schedule) and you are often left with regret (if only we had...).

I must add a section of commentary on the subject of expectations. The difference between encouragement and pressure is unnecessary expectations. We must realize that our children are unique creations from the hand of the Almighty God. A doctor's son does not have to become a doctor. The son of an athletic father does not have to be good at sports—he may not even like sports. The daughter of a teacher may not like to teach. The son of a pastor may not like to preach. The daughter of a lawyer may never study law. The son of a dentist may never touch a jaw.

Please allow your children to choose their own areas of interest and teach them to thank God for their unique gifts and abilities. "And whatever you do, whether in word or deed, do it all in the name of the Lord Jesus, *giving thanks* to God the Father through Him" (Col. 3:17; emphasis added).

Unnecessary expectations will only lead to disappointment, disillusionment, and discouragement for both the parent and the child. Love, support, and encouragement will lead to acceptance and joy. Parents, allow your Creator to mold and shape each child; remember, they are to become Christ-like, not parent-like.

16

We Must Learn to Listen!

WHEN A LITTLE CHILD IS born, parents can hardly wait to hear their child talk. We focus our energy and we spend hours teaching our children how to talk. When do we as parents teach our children how to listen? As parents, we often times complain to our children that they didn't listen—but did we ever teach them how to listen?

Listening is not a natural process that develops over time. Hearing may be, but not true listening. Unfortunately, this lack of verbal comprehension often goes undetected and penetrates our adult relationships. Many adults would rather assume than ask.

King Saul is a perfect example of one who heard but did not listen. In 1 Samuel 13, a story is told in which Saul was to *wait for Samuel to come* and offer burnt and fellowship offerings. Samuel would come in seven days. King Saul heard *burnt offering in seven days*, which is exactly what he did in Samuel's absence. Verses 13 and 14 record Samuel's response to King Saul:

You have acted foolishly, Samuel said. You have not kept the command the LORD your God gave you; if you had, He would have established your kingdom over Israel for all time. But now your kingdom will not endure; the LORD has sought out a man after His own heart and appointed him leader of His people, because you have not kept the LORD's command.

King Saul heard what he wanted to hear. He did not listen and obey! Listening is the first step, our obedient response is the completion of the process; however, we can't complete the process until we listen. James 1:22 states, "Do not merely listen to the word, and so deceive yourselves. Do what it says." First John 4:6 says, "We are from God, and whoever knows God listens to us; but whoever is not from God does not listen to us. This is how we recognize the Spirit of truth and the spirit of falsehood."

Following are the results of a survey I gave to high school students in a church youth group I was teaching:

- Ninety-six percent stated they loved their birth mother and birth father
- Ninety-two percent felt loved by their birth parents
- Forty-one percent were living in divorced homes
- Ninety-six percent seldom or never read the Bible together as a family
- Ninety-six percent seldom or never prayed together as a family

- Sixty-three percent did not attend church together as a family
- Nineteen percent often spent time alone with their parents
- Fifty-five percent had good to great communication with their mother
- Thirty-two percent had good to great communication with their father
- Forty-eight percent stated both parents were confessing Christians

The results from this survey led me to the following conclusions: our high school group feels love for and from their parents; they face the fear of parental divorce; they spend virtually no time in prayer or scripture reading with their parents; they do not attend church together as a family on a regular basis; they find it easier to communicate with their mother than with their father.

Next, I wanted to see if those who answered that both their parents were confessing Christians (48 percent) changed the above conclusions.

- Parental divorce? *Yes*—thirty-three percent
- Prayer or Scripture reading? *Seldom or never*—ninety-two percent
- Family church attendance together? *Yes*—forty-two percent
- Communication with mother: *Great or good*—fifty-eight percent
- Communication with father: *Great or good*—thirty-six percent

The same conclusions are valid in the Christian home. Now granted, these are high school students and not elementary age children; however, I think the conclusions are still important to acknowledge and comprehend. If our elementary-aged children are not praying with us, reading scripture with us and attending church with us today, they are certainly less likely to do so in high school tomorrow. If we want our communication to be good to great in high school, we need to ensure it is great at the elementary age. The principle of the Sower is very real for parents—we reap what we sow. Meditate upon the words from the song "Cats in the Cradle" and listen to the lament in the father's voice.

How would your children respond to these questions? Most fathers are less accessible to their children (number of hours per week) than mothers are. This means that these fathers must make a greater effort to listen and ask questions. Yes, I said ask questions! Mom: one of the best things you can do is to encourage/schedule one on one time for your husband to spend with each child. These daddy/daughter date nights and father/son outings are pivotal for their relationships. And while you are at it, mom, schedule one on one times for yourself as well. One of Caleb's favorite memories is attending an Oakland A's baseball game with his mom when he was eight years old. He caught his first foul ball that day—while mom was in the bathroom (true story).

Our family is making a habit of sitting down for dinner together (with the television and radio turned off) and discussing the same two questions every night. Question 1: What is the *best* thing that happened to you today? Our children love sharing the most exciting event of each day. Question 2: what is the *worst* thing that happened to you today? The smile may leave the lips of the person sharing; however, each family member knows they have teammates sitting at the table with them ready to support (prayer, hug, possible solution).

It is absolutely critical that this time of sharing be respected and open. If critical comments or judgment follow this sharing time, the children will *learn* to stop sharing openly and honestly. Some issues require parental privacy (away from other siblings) and some issues require discipline (confession does not negate consequences). The family members will get a good feel for what is proper to share during this time and wise parents will defer inappropriate conversations to a more private arena.

I am pleasantly surprised by how important/fun it is to our children that they listen to Mom and Dad's best and worst events of the day. This simple exercise leads to teachable moments for the children, opportunities for family prayer, further discussions for Mom and Dad (after the kids go to bed), and a growing sense of *family*: teammates committed to relational growth and common objectives.

Parents, how can we identify with the pressures our children face at school and elsewhere if we don't know them? What better way is there to show that we care than by elevating their concerns and fears to our Heavenly Father? If our children do not hear our prayers and see us reading His word, what message do we send? If we tell our children to attend church but find ourselves too busy to accompany them, what message do we send?

Why do our children find it difficult to communicate with us? Let's personalize this question! Why does my child find it difficult to communicate with me? Do I not listen very well? Do I seem uncaring or unapproachable? Do I condemn or judge them every time they open up with me? Do I give fluff answers like "Don't worry, be happy!"?

Learning how to actively listen can dramatically change your relationship with any child. Simply remember to use basic communication skills like the following.

Face the speaker
Be aware of your body language
Maintain eye contact at all times
Ask questions if you do not understand
Restate their feelings to show you understand
Encourage the speaker to express their feelings

Do not be quick to judge your child's feelings or feel like you have to solve *their* problem for *them*. Help *them* work through *their* feelings and help *them* develop a solution to *their* problems. Please remember that their fears and concerns are real to them no matter how trivial they may seem to you.

Our response should be like that of our Heavenly Father! "Cast all your anxiety on Him because He cares for you" (1 Pet. 5:7). "Do not be anxious about anything, but in everything, by prayer and petition, with thanksgiving, present your requests to God. And the peace of God, which transcends all understanding, will guard your hearts and your minds in Christ Jesus" (Phil. 4:6–7).

Our Heavenly Father knows how to listen! He doesn't judge our fears, He calms them; He doesn't ignore our concerns, He comforts them; He isn't too busy to listen to our worries, He meets us where we are; He doesn't solve our problems for us, He guides us through them. Listening is a primary act of the Holy Spirit! He is our comforter, our counselor, and our guide!

Romans 8:26–27 says it this way: "In the same way, the Spirit helps us in our weakness. We do not know what we ought to pray for, but the Spirit Himself intercedes for us with groans that words cannot express. And He who searches our hearts knows the mind of the Spirit, because the Spirit intercedes for the saints in accordance with God's will."

Our communication must become more than being available and willing to help our children with their fears, worries, and concerns. We must show our children that we enjoy them! Ask them about their interests. When they get excited, get excited with them. Be there for their ball games or concerts. Take them away to the mountains and talk to them about our loving Creator. Take them to the beach and talk to them about the power of God. Ask them what they would like to do and where they would like to go (within reason) and just listen to them talk. You will become amazed at how simple fun events can open up lines for more intimate communication down the road.

When Caleb was ten years old, I took him on a one-week bus trip through the Mid-West where we saw professional baseball games each night. We talked about God's purpose for sex and dating on the shores of Lake Michigan.

Later, when he was thirteen, I took him away to Oakland for a weekend series of A's games, and using the Focus on the Family Passport to Purity kit, we continued the conversation about God's purpose for sex and dating. Regina scheduled similar trips with our girls when they turned thirteen. We need to listen and we need to be intentional about the message and we need to show interest.

Ask yourself, *whom do I open up with and why?* The *why* probably includes trust and freedom from judgment and shows a real interest.

My father began family devotions with my brother and I when I was thirteen years old and they continued every night (even during college breaks) until I left home to marry at age twenty-three. I learned during these devotions that a relationship with Jesus Christ was personal and that He desired my heart every day. I knew that every night I would have my concerns lifted up in prayer with my family. This family devotion time not only assisted me in developing my own personal relationship with Jesus, it also helped me in developing a personal relationship with my father, my mother, and my brother. Listening is not an activity, it is a way of life.

Parents, how can we identify with the pressures our children face at school and elsewhere if we don't know them?

17

Parent for Outcomes

WHY DO WE NEED TO parent? Because we have been blessed with an incredible gift from our Heavenly Father that has some assembly required. We need to view each child as an investment that will produce righteous living with loving kindness. Like the Parable of the Talents in Matt. 25, we long to receive God's gift, invest wisely and hear our Master say: "Well done, good and faithful servant! Come and share your master's happiness!"

I want to encourage you to parent for the following three outcomes:

Self-Confident – Joshua 1:9 "Have I not commanded you? Be strong and courageous. Do not be terrified; do not be discouraged, for the Lord your God will be with you wherever you go."

The number one question my wife and I were asked about our children was: How did your children develop such self-confidence at a young age? The funny thing is neither Regina nor I were self-confident as a youth. We were asked so many times that we started paying attention to what we were doing. Here is what we discovered.

We placed a high value on open and honest communication. We asked many questions. We shared openly about our success and failure. We encouraged trying new things. We taught that a failed attempt today is valuable tomorrow. We taught that "suffering produces perseverance; perseverance, character; and character, hope. And hope does not disappoint us because God poured out His love into our hearts by the Holy Spirit, whom He has given us" (Romans 5: 3-5).

We encouraged and exhorted each child to serve on mission trips, attend church camps & youth groups, join multiple athletic teams, enjoy music and the arts, learn how to write creatively, learn how to speak publicly and learn how to think critically before they began high school. We encouraged them "to live self-controlled, upright and godly lives" (Titus 2:12) and that "God did not give us a spirit of timidity, but a spirit of power, of love and of self-discipline" (2 Timothy 1:7).

We taught each child to compete to win – according to the rules (2 Timothy 2:5); while giving thanks to Jesus – in both word and deed (Colossians 3:17); and by speaking and serving for the glory of God (1 Peter 4:11).

Caleb was cut from his junior high soccer team in 7th grade and started for the first-place team in 8th grade; he was cut from Frosh/Soph high school basketball as a sophomore and made the Varsity team his junior and senior year. He took each temporary failure as an opportunity to practice and get better. He still coaches basketball today.

Rebekah scored 25 goals her freshman and sophomore year of JV soccer and decided to try-out for the School musical, instead of playing Varsity soccer her junior year. This is despite not being in the drama class and being completely unknown to the drama teacher (who had most of these students for two or three years already). Oh, by the way, she wanted the lead role. Guess who played Sandy in Grease that year? Not a surprise to her parents, she shared the lead in our Church Christmas Musical as a 4th grader—competing against 6th graders. For good measure, she made the starting Varsity track team in multiple events her senior year.

Sarah excelled in all her sports, especially soccer and softball. Unfortunately, both sports crossed over in high school so she chose to continue with soccer. Her junior year in high school she convinced the softball coach to let her try-out (mid-season and after not playing competitively for two years—and also unknown to this coach). She made the team—which was ranked in the state of CA. Mom and Dad found out about this after the try-out. She was confident enough to approach the coach on her own.

Our children have been working summers since the age of fourteen. Most of the jobs required zero help from Regina and I. They never took a summer off. They learned a strong work-ethic, they learned how to effectively communicate, and they grew in confidence with each success and learned failure.

We were not helicopter parents! When our children had issues with teachers or students or youth leaders, they shared with us, we strategized and *they* carried it out. We did not apologize for them! If their behavior hurt others, *they* apologized. They understood the links between values, behavior, accountability and consequences. We did not baby our children and we did not set low expectations. We taught them to dream big within the perfect Will of God.

1 John 2:28 states: "And now, dear children, continue in Him, so that when He appears we may be confident and unashamed before Him at His coming." Our children were taught at the earliest age they were fearfully and wonderfully made in the image of God (Psalm 139:14), that God had a wonderful plan for their life – giving them hope and a future (Jeremiah 29:11), that they belong to God (Romans 1:6) and that they can do everything through Christ Jesus who gives them strength (Philippians 4:13).

Responsible – Proverbs 22:6 "Train a child in the way he should go, and when he is old he will not turn from it."

I believe that values drive commitment; commitment determines responsible behavior; and responsible behavior reveals our testimony. Regina and I believe in parenting with purpose – with both love and logic. We believe parents are commanded to train, equip and encourage each child to glorify God, utilizing the talents and passions God uniquely blessed and wired each child with. This requires each parent to become a student of each child.

The Holden Home had several rules that were clearly defined and communicated. It started with our values. We value the Word of God, relationships, education, laughing, teamwork, the fruit of the Spirit and acts of service. Our values helped us prioritize our commitments – church and devotional time as a family, enjoying time with family and friends, saving money for college, watching comedy shows and movies together, attending one another's activities and cheering wildly, developing godly character and serving inside and outside our community.

Our values helped us as parents determine activities. Our children were actively involved in our church AWANA program from Kindergarten through eighth grade; they were engaged in Sunday school classes and small groups from K-12; they were required to maintain a 3.0 or better in school (with good comments in attitude and sportsmanship); they were required to be involved in a school and/ or outside school activity (sports, music, service, etc.); they were given money to manage and taught to tithe, save and spend wisely; they were required to work outside the home during summers from age 14 on; they were assigned household chores and held accountable for completing them on time with excellence; they were given pets to care for; and they joyfully participated in "family" time – especially annual vacations to Lake Tahoe with extended family and away to places like Disneyland or Disney World.

Our priorities helped during times of conflict. Our children all played on travel sports teams; however, they rarely missed church on Sundays or youth group on Wednesday nights – the higher value was church (we, unfortunately, watched many other children struggle later with their Christian values when the athletic team was placed as the higher priority). Our children were not allowed the extra activities if it took significant time away from their church commitments or if they were unable to keep a 3.0 in school.

For those who worry about overextending our children with activities and commitments, I acknowledge that each child is unique. I also acknowledge that often times it is truly the parent who does not want to commit to the time it takes to drive and cheer each child on. Sarah in junior high was on a church basketball team, school softball team and club soccer team – at the same time - while keeping her church commitments and academic requirements. She understood the priorities and made it work. What she did not do was spend much time sitting in front of a television or on her phone. In fact, all the way through college, her GPA was always best when she was involved in a team sport.

Caleb played baseball, basketball, soccer and tennis non-stop through high school and rarely missed youth group and only once missed the 3.0 for a short period of time. He played five different intra-mural sports in college and graduated cum laude. Rebekah played sports, piano, led youth group worship from 6th grade on, taught herself to play the guitar, participated in numerous musicals and graduated valedictorian in high school and summa cum laude in college. And she planned a wedding and was married to her college sweetheart two weeks after graduating in three and a half years.

I must remind you that Regina and I are far from remarkable. Our children are better students and servants than we are. We simply taught them what to value, how to prioritize these values and supported them with opportunities to find their passion and discover their gifts. We spent much time driving our children to their events and often had to divide our time together to make it all work – and you know what? We would do it all again in a heartbeat!

These activities taught our children how to be *responsible* with their time, how to give their best effort and gave them a platform to share their faith. It is impossible to put into words the joy Regina and I felt as we watched our children invite their non-Christian teammates to church and into our home, sharing their testimony in word and deed. God used our children to help bring other children into His kingdom – this does not happen if our kids remain inside watching TV and playing video games all day.

We taught each child the value of *stewardship* – it all belongs to God; the value of *surrendering* - our will to His will; and the need to serve God and others – by becoming His hands and feet.

Servant Leaders - Ephesians 6:7 "Serve wholeheartedly, as if you were serving the Lord, not men."

I believe God has called us to be leaders: fishers of men (Matt. 4:19), disciple-makers (Matt. 28:19) and Ambassadors for Christ (2 Cor. 5:20). The first principle of leadership is in knowing whom and how to follow. The whom is Jesus and the how is wholehearted.

One does not need to be an outgoing, extroverted, highly gifted individual to become a leader – just look at Jesus' disciples: uneducated fishermen, a tax collector, a Zealot and a traitor. Jesus says Come and follow me and I will *make* you…

As young, inexperienced parents, Regina and I watched the older children in our church and spoke with parents we admired. We discovered that children learning and developing ownership for godly *convictions* at an early age – making their faith their own, not their parent's faith – developed into teenagers who were able to stand against temptation and lead others toward the goodness of God.

They understood the value of both obedience and forgiveness. They understood their responsibility was to share their story and to allow the Holy Spirit to harvest.

One Christmas season our family served as bell ringers for the Salvation Army; we served together at City Team ministries serving the homeless; we participated in numerous Church plays; and we served together in child-care at church. Our children spent time volunteering as Coaches, worship leaders, teachers, referees, child-care, elder-care and assisting children with special needs.

Our ultimate goal is to be with Jesus and have Him say to us: "Well done, good and faithful servant!" (Matt. 25:21). As parents, we need to teach our children how to be led by the Holy Spirit (Romans 8:14) and when leading, to govern diligently (Romans 12:8). This requires us as parents to ensure we are being led by the Holy Spirit and are governing diligently.

I have observed and learned that the greatest ability to lead is our availability and willingness to serve. I have been blessed with numerous leadership opportunities at my church, my workplace and my community – and I have rarely, if ever, initiated the conversation. I have learned to prepare my heart and my schedule to lead and God opens the doors of opportunity. At one church I spent three years simply directing parking cars in between services. Whatever God wants!

Regina became an AWANA leader and ultimately was asked to be the Commander. She became a Stephen minister and was asked to lead the women as the Coordinator. Caleb was asked to be head coach of his church softball team (in his early twenties, leading men in their thirties and forties) the second season he played at a church he just started attending. Rebekah was asked to lead the greater Sacramento area for Day of Prayer, working alongside KLOVE radio. Sarah was appointed captain of her soccer team that won state and in high school was voted in as team chaplain – at a public school in Texas.

These are just some of the leadership roles accepted – all of them came from people watching their lives and asking them to lead. It begins with a heart to love people and a willingness to serve others. Leadership is influence. Servant Leaders understand the role of the leader is to serve those we lead. We train, we equip, we encourage, we promote, we support and we wash their feet. Sounds a lot like Jesus; sounds a lot like parenting!

We want to develop children who grow to become thermostats (affecting their surroundings by controlling their environment around them), rather than thermometers (being affected *by* their surroundings, causing them to rise or fall). We want our children pro-active and leading, not reactive and responding. Servant Leaders are called to serve, not to be served (Matt. 20:25-28); to be patient, not impatient (Eph. 4:1-3); to be humble, not proud (Phil. 2:3-8); and to teach, rather than be quarrelsome (2 Tim. 2:23, 24).

Our goal as parents is to introduce each child to Jesus, to model godly living by setting an example in "speech, in life, in love, in faith and in purity" (1 Tim. 4:12), and to help our babies grow into self-confident, responsible, servant-leaders by the time they leave our home! This requires an investment of our time, treasure and talents. I am here to tell you that every second, every dime and every drop of sweat is worth it.

The outcome produces young adults who are able to go away to college and make wise choices; who are able to interview for jobs and responsible enough to keep them; who are prepared to develop authentic relationships; who are ready, willing and able to leave a lasting, positive impression in our society; and who are driven to further the kingdom of God.

During Caleb's senior year in college, he wrote me the following letter, placed it in a sports-themed hand-made frame and gave it to me on father's day. It brought me to tears of joy and it still resides above my desk at work today.

> *Thank You For:*
> *Teaching me sports and being my coach.*
> *Being so generous with your time and money.*
> *All of the family vacations and the trips for just the two of us. Taking Jay Buckley's baseball trip of the Midwest is still one of the best things I have ever done. Going to the Rose Bowl is also a memory I love and will always treasure.*
> *Being the greatest role model, and showing how a husband and father should treat his wife and kids.*
> *Speaking into my life spiritually and praying for me every day. I especially want*

to thank you for calling me out before Hume Lake my senior year because you caused me to think about my relationship with God. Without your words of wisdom, I do not know how long it would have taken me to make my faith my own.

Always inviting conversation and the amount of fun you are to hang out and talk with. I absolutely love how we joke around with each other.

Believing in me and supporting me in whatever I do. I know you always have my back and want nothing more than to see me succeed. I so appreciate how you have never stopped coaching me, even when you are no longer coaching me in sports.

Being my hero.

Repeatedly telling me you love me, even though I do not say it back near as often as I should. So Dad,

I LOVE YOU!

18

This World Is Not Our Home!

WHILE READING THE SCRIPTURES, SEARCHING for Bible verses that teach about parenting, I discovered an interesting passage that I believe applies very well. The passage is entitled "Treasures in Jars of Clay" and can be found in 2 Corinthians chapter 4.

How are our children like Treasures in Jars of Clay? Well, clay can be easily molded and shaped when it is young and impressionable, like our children. After it hardens and sets, it is difficult to reshape or change. Our children's first twelve years are critical during this shaping process. Clay also becomes more fragile over time and chips easily where the quality and quantity of the clay is lacking. In other words, the more clay used and the greater the attention to structure, the more solid the clay becomes and is able to withstand harsh treatment.

Balance again is the key! We do not want to enwrap our children in steel where they cannot feel any pain and thus be unable to feel compassion; unable to experience hurt, where our greatest growth often times takes place. Similarly, we do not want to store our children in glass jars that become easily broken at the sign of any kind of trouble or persecution. No, we want our children crafted in clay, where they can experience the "chips and nicks" in life yet still be able to serve a useful purpose.

Fathers, the Bible tells us not to "exasperate" (Eph. 6:4) or "embitter" (Col. 3:21) our children. We need to raise offspring who are excited and desirous of serving Jesus. Please do not put upon your children a heavy yoke of unnecessary expectations and needless stress—too many of our Christian youth today find themselves unmotivated and too tired to make a difference in this world.

Having not enough scars can be just as damaging as having too many scars. We need to raise children who will carry on the work of Jesus Christ; children, who respect the marks upon their Savior's hands and feet; children, who can be chipped and nicked without breaking. We need to raise children who are willing to stand at the gate of hell and give directions to heaven.

I would like to return to our passage in 2 Corinthians chapter four, and I would like to focus on verses 16–18 (emphasis added) which state,

> Therefore we do not lose heart. Though outwardly we are wasting away, yet inwardly we are being renewed day by day. *For our light and momentary troubles are achieving for us an eternal glory that far outweighs them all.* So we fix our eyes not on what is seen, but on what is unseen.

> For what is seen is temporary, but what is
> unseen is eternal.

Our children are eternal treasures from God! They will cause us light and momentary troubles; they will require us to sacrifice. But the eternal glory (salvation for them and eternal fellowship with them for us) far outweighs any temporary struggles we may experience.

Fathers, do not lose heart. The Holy Spirit will renew your strength and joy day by day, and He will enable you to raise godly children.

Mothers, do not despair. The Holy Spirit will gird you with a peace and calm that surpasses all understanding, and He will enable you to raise children filled with compassion and love in a world that so desperately needs it.

The key is for us to fix our eyes on that which is unseen; that which is eternal! We may see a wild two-year-old that only knows how to say *no*, but within that little child dwells a future leader who will teach others to say *no* to sin and *yes* to Jesus. We may see a quiet four-year-old that hates the outdoors and loves to read books, but soon that four-year-old will grow up and begin writing books about Jesus that will encourage people into having a personal relationship with Him. We may see our seven-year-old as an overly sensitive crybaby, but in time, that crybaby will become a doctor who will use that sensitivity to heal the wounds of others.

We must learn to see our children as eternal creations; we must learn to see our children through our Heavenly Father's eyes. The sacrifices made today may reap eternal rewards tomorrow. The little child who lives in your house is more than just flesh and bones—he/she is eternal. Joyfully conceived and beautifully born; eagerly awaiting an introduction to their loving Creator and Savior, Jesus Christ. When we view raising children through the perspective glass of eternity, what sacrifice is too great to make? What service is too hard to perform? What treasure is too great to lay aside?

We may examine our life and label our self "sinner." Our Heavenly Father erases the word *sinner* and replaces it with "saved by grace." Isaiah 64:8 says, "Yet, O LORD, you are our Father. We are the clay, you are the potter; we are all the work of your hand."

Parents, no matter how poor of a father or mother you may have been in the past, today you can choose to change. Our Heavenly Father has entrusted us with young, fresh, impressionable clay that we are to mold into His image. We are not expected to produce a perfect product—our Heavenly Father will do that—we are simply asked to help shape and to help present the clay to the Master Potter. The best way to accomplish this is by allowing the Master Potter to mold us into His image first. I encourage you to take some time right now and pray to your Heavenly Father. Thank Him for the treasure He has entrusted you with and seek His guidance and assistance in presenting the treasure back to Him.

Therefore, I urge you, brothers, in view of God's mercy, to offer your bodies as living sacrifices, holy and pleasing to

God—this is your spiritual act of worship. Do not conform any longer to the pattern of this world, but be transformed by the renewing of your mind. Then you will be able to test and approve what God's will is—His good, pleasing and perfect will. (Rom. 12:1–2).

Epilogue

THANK YOU FOR TAKING THIS Parenting journey with me. My journey started over 25 years ago and it still continues today. My Adult children taught me another lesson this past Christmas: the importance of *thoughtfulness* & *generosity*. As we left our hectic personal lives and gathered together for family time back in our nest- now even more precious with a son-in-law and daughter-in-law joining us—I was blessed and awed by the thoughtfulness and generosity of my children. Each gift was carefully crafted or purchased with intent and intimacy. Dedicated time was spent sharing memories and building new ones. Laughter and Listening ruled the week we spent together.

I was reminded that thoughtfulness and generosity covers our time, our treasure and our talents—and does not require a large sum of money. I was reminded that even though Regina and I have an empty nest on most days, we are blessed to have "one another" and to have children who enjoy coming home to visit. I was reminded that my family continues to grow—incredible in-laws and someday grandchildren. I was reminded that my journey continues.

In 1 Timothy 6: 17-19 (emphasis added), Paul reminds us to place our hope in God, who lavishes us with everything we need for our enjoyment. Paul then drops this wonderful prompt that I believe applies perfectly for parents: "Command them to do good, to be rich in good deeds, and to be *generous* and willing to share. In this way they will lay up treasure for themselves as a firm foundation for the coming age, so that they may take hold of the life that is truly life."

Thoughtful and generous parents produce thoughtful and generous children, who become thoughtful and generous parents, who will produce thoughtful and generous grandchildren. We serve a very thoughtful and generous God!

Our children trust us to love and provide for them, and we trust our Heavenly Father to assist us with this awesome responsibility and privilege. I am discovering that as a parent, sometimes all I can do is trust. Thank God that I have someone to share my fears and concerns with. Someone to share my joy and excitement with. That someone is my Heavenly Father and His precious Son, Jesus Christ.

What I enjoyed most about being a parent with young children was knowing two things: my children *needed* me and my children *trusted* me. When my children wanted to play, it was me that they sought; whenever they fell down and got hurt, again they came to me; whenever they wanted to be rocked or have a book read to them, they counted on me to meet their desire. They were dependent upon me in so many different ways—no pride, no shame, no fear— they just came to me.

Our Heavenly Father seeks the same from each of us. He feels tremendous joy whenever we come to Him with our needs and wants—when we learn to trust Him—

when we learn to become dependent upon Him. He created us (in His image), He nurtures and protects us (in the shadow of His wings), and He loves us (unconditionally and everlasting).

So...Why Parent? Because:

1) It is your calling from God to do so as a mom or dad
2) It produces long-term, eternal relationships of family
3) It enables us to better understand our relationship with our Heavenly Father
4) It makes the decision of choosing Jesus easier for our grandchildren
5) If you don't, the World will!

It is my sincere hope that this book may have somehow stirred the embers of joy in your heart for raising children. Nothing—absolutely nothing—will assist you in becoming a good, joyful, and calm parent more than a solid personal relationship with Jesus Christ. Allow our Heavenly Father to guide you along your parenting journey. *Be glad and be calm!*

Are You?

Children are a heritage from the LORD,
Knitted and crafted to be adored.
Laughter and singing should fill every room,
When children are born to each bride and groom.
Are you glad to be a dad?
Are you calm to be a mom?

I wish tranquil for Jill and joy for Roy,
As they love and rear each girl and boy.
I wish peace for Reese and jolly for Holly,
As they play lots of sports and dress-up with Dolly.
Are you glad to be a dad?
Are you calm to be a mom?

Have fun with each child. Don't live with regret.
Prepare to get wild or silly or wet.
Grab a ball, read a book, or go for a walk.
Stay up for hours learning to talk.
Are you glad to be a dad?
Are you calm to be a mom?

Time goes by so fast, so why do you wait?
Go on have a blast, before it's too late.
When your nest becomes quiet through passage of time,
Remember my words in this simple rhyme.
Are you glad to be a dad?
Are you calm to be a mom?

Now this is the end of my little poem.
Grab the hand, kiss the cheek of your child at home.
And always remember to thank God above,
For sending His child in showing us *love*.
Be glad! Be calm!

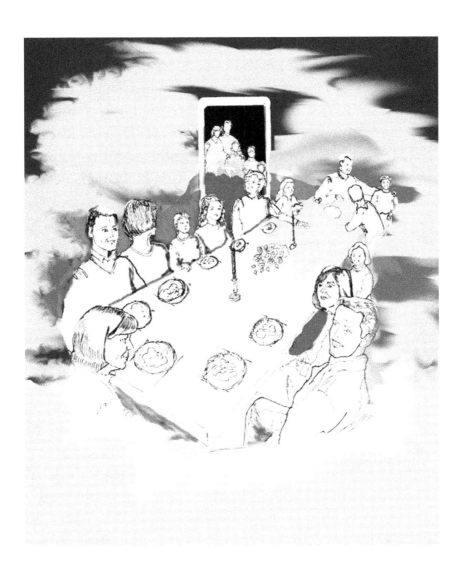

About the Author

DAVID HOLDEN HAS BEEN MARRIED thirty years to his beautiful wife, Regina, and is the father of four children: Caleb (27), Rebekah (25), Joshua (deceased), and Sarah (21). He began writing this book shortly after the birth of his first son. He is now finally ready to share what he learned.

He graduated with his BS from Biola University (business management) and with his BA from William Jessup University in Bible and Theology. Years later, he received his masters in organizational leadership through Biola University in 2010.

David is the vice president for Radiation Detection Company, where he manages human resources and organizational development. He actively serves as a deacon and teacher at First Baptist Church, Georgetown in Georgetown, Texas. He does some on-line adjunct teaching for William Jessup University.

The following summarizes his parenting heart: "In no way was I or am I a perfect parent, but God has blessed my family as I learned His purpose for my parenting. All my children elected to minor in Bible, are actively serving the LORD, and are in healthy, godly, relationships (my oldest two are married to college sweethearts and my youngest is currently engaged to her college sweetheart). I am not a pastor, missionary, or world-famous evangelist—I am a simple Christian dad who studied *why* God parents us and did my best to *learn* as a *son*, and to *apply* as a *dad—calmly, with great joy*—God's parenting principles for His children who He trusted my wife and I to help raise."

David believes with all his heart that young parents today need to be encouraged *and* need to be reminded to enjoy the process. This is not a how-to-parent book; this is a *why-to-parent* book. He has included a devotional aspect to this book for those who want to use it as a personal devotional or in a parenting class setting.

He would love to hear your stories about the parenting journey you are on and if this book helped encourage you along that path. You may email him at gladdad2018@ gmail.com.

Study Guide

Part I Chapter 1: Marriage Requires...

The Foundation of Marriage

1. All marriages face _____
2. _____ and _____ are the two primary ingredients for a healthy marriage.
3. A strong foundation is needed both before and after _____.
4. Children need to see our commitment to _____, _____, and _____.

The Fundamentals of Marriage

1. The four fundamentals of marriage are
   a. _____
   b. _____
   c. _____
   d. _____

2. Communication requires both _____ and _____.

3. Communication is only as good as it is framed in
   _____.
4. We need to _____ before we speak.
5. Marriage is a _____ relationship.
6. In spite of changes the _____
   _____ of our mate remains_____.
7. The ability to say _____ is an absolute
   must for a healthy marriage.
8. Love is a _____.
9. Companionship must be the result of _____
   _____.
10. Our relationship as husband and wife impacts our
    _____ view of marriage.

Action Steps: Do as many as you can.

What will I do specifically to

1. keep my marriage fresh and exciting?

2. demonstrate my family's commitment to Christ?

3. improve my communication with my spouse and
   children?

4. demonstrate that I am trustworthy?

5. forgive my spouse and/or children?

6. show love to my spouse and children in tangible ways?

7. spend more "alone" time with my spouse?

Part I Chapter 2 Life Hasn't Changed, Roles Have

Church

1. Church is a _____
   of God's kingdom that is being established and
   used by God for His glory through His people.
2. As our knowledge and understanding change, so
   do our _____.
3. Our family should imitate a _____
   _____.

Family

1. We must focus our _____ on our
   spouse and family.
2. Our primary objective is to enjoy our _____
   with God and with one another.
3. Relationships are _____, professions
   are _____.

Work

1. Our business world needs men and women with
   a. _____
   b. _____
   c. _____

2. Parents need to choose time with family and
   _____ God to honor that commitment.

3. Our calling is to _____ our spouse and to raise our children in the _____ and _____ of the Lord.

School

1. When we stop studying and learning, we start _____.
2. We must remain _____ so the Holy Spirit can mold us and teach us how to best love and respect Christ.
3. Children enjoy learning when parents _____ in the learning process with them.
4. God has equipped us with a natural parenting intuition and has given us the _____ and His _____ to help us.
5. Parents must continue to learn so that we will be properly equipped and able to teach and train our family in the way of _____.

Action Steps: Do as many as you can.

What will I do specifically to

1. build a strong family ministry?

2. teach my children how to give?

3. focus my identity on my spouse and children?

4. balance work, family, and service to honor God?

5. fulfill my eternal calling?

6. proactively teach my children to enjoy learning?

Part I Chapter 3 Divorce from a Kid's Perspective

1. God _____ divorce.
2. _____ are often overlooked when a divorce is chosen.
3. Divorce is the _____ to a death in the family.
4. Divorce is a breach of trust that hampers the parent–child _____.
5. Divorce destroys a child's _____ _____ for a sense of belonging.
6. Children of divorced parents need a solid _____ youth group.
7. Divorced parents need a solid _____ support group.
8. Children need to see Mom and Dad in love with each other and _____ together.
9. No marriage is beyond _____, for in Christ Jesus, all things are possible.
10. Glad to be a dad and calm to be a mom begins with _____ to be a husband and _____ to be a wife.

Action Steps: Do as many as you can.

What will I do specifically to

1. let my children see my spouse and I in love with each other?

2. deal with marital problems as they occur?

3. support parents and children that have experienced divorce?

Part II Chapter 4 Self-Control

1. The first goal of parenting is to have _____ give way to _____; and _____ give way to _____.
2. Children learn _____ behavior by what they are _____.
3. God has given me His _____ to communicate what is _____ behavior for me.
4. God has given me His _____ to dwell within me and to remind me of my commitment to _____.
5. As I allow God's Spirit to fill me, I develop the fruit of _____ and am able to say *no* to _____ and *yes* to _____.
6. The more _____ I develop in my life, the more _____ I can help my child develop in his/her life.
7. Catch your children doing things _____!

Action Steps: Do as many as you can.

What will I do specifically to

1. teach my children what behavior is acceptable and not acceptable?

2. become a student of God's Word and be filled daily with His Spirit?

3. identify the areas in my life that need self-control?

4. help my children develop self-control?

5. praise my children for acceptable behavior and godly choices?

Part II Chapter 5 Incarnation

1. Young children like to _____ their parent's _____.
2. As a Christian, I am called to _____ the behavior of _____.
3. Disciple means "_____."
4. We can _____ to Jesus because He can _____ to us.
5. As parents, we need to become _____ _____ to our children.
6. As parents, we need to become _____ _____ to our children.
7. As parents, we need to _____ our children at their level of _____.

Action Steps: Do as many as you can.

What will I do specifically to

1. intentionally model the behavior of Jesus to my children?

2. serve my children?

3. better understand the role of Jesus as my merciful and faithful high priest (Heb. 2:14–18) and how that applies to my parenting?

4. support other leaders in the life of my children— teachers, coaches, pastors, etc.?

5. meet my children at their level of growth?

Part II Chapter 6 Security and Trust

1. As my _____ increases, so does my _____ and _____ increase.
2. Children are born into this world with a natural sense of _____.
3. By adulthood, many people have less _____ and _____ in their lives.
4. Parents also have _____ needs.
5. A _____ with Jesus Christ is the only _____ that will provide constant _____ and _____ without fail.
6. We should be striving for _____ instead of _____.
7. We must make our home a place of _____ and _____ for our family.

Action Steps: Do as many as you can.

What will I do specifically to

1. better understand and identify my security needs?

2. teach my children to trust God with their security needs?

3. better understand how hope becomes an anchor for our soul (Heb. 6:19)?

4. become more dependent upon the daily presence of the Holy Spirit in my life?

5. ensure my home is a place of security, trust and comfort for my family?

Part II Chapter 7 Love

1. Parents need to show _____ love and _____ to their children.
2. Choosing to love is a _____ behavior for a child.
3. Choosing to love is a _____ behavior for an adult.
4. God is _____.
5. _____ love teaches our children that _____ are more important than effort.
6. _____ love teaches our children that _____ is more important than _____.
7. _____ can learn much about love by watching their _____.

Action Steps: Do as many as you can.

What will I do specifically to

1. show unconditional love and acceptance to each child?

2. identify actions/behavior in my life that may teach my children my love is conditional?

3. teach the importance of developing godly character to my children?

4. verbally express my unconditional love for each
   child?

5. build my home upon the rock of unconditional
   love and acceptance?

Part II Chapter 8 Image

1. Mankind alone is _____ in the _____ of God.
2. Mankind is still in the _____ of God after the _____.
3. *Image* goes much deeper than _____ resemblance.
4. Our _____ nature desires for us to _____ the image of God.
5. As we _____ the image of God, we become _____ to the image of Christ.
6. Children learn through _____.
7. As parents we are _____.

Action Steps: Do as many as you can.

What will I do specifically to

1. recognize I am created in the image of God and of my parents and that my children are created in my image?

2. develop my spiritual nature over my sinful nature and teach my children how?

3. become conformed to the image of Christ?

4. help my children learn positive lessons through observation?

5. better understand my parenting role as a Mediator?

Part II Chapter 9 Discipline and Repentance

1. God has blessed my child with a _____ and _____ personality.
2. Parents need to _____ each child to _____ the _____ will.
3. Start with a _____ line of discipline during the _____ years.
4. Discipline over _____ that matter to _____.
5. Parents need to take the _____ necessary to _____ proper discipline.
6. Discipline because you _____ the child and desire to _____ acceptable behavior.
7. Teaching _____ encompasses far more than _____.

Action Steps: Do as many as you can.

What will I do specifically to

1. ensure my will matches God's will so my discipline is His standard?

2. learn which discipline methods work best for each child?

3. communicate my plan to reduce restrictions and protection as my child demonstrates responsibility and self-control?

4. free up time in my schedule to allow me to administer proper discipline?

Part II Chapter 10 One Another

1. Each child is _____gifted with talents, personalities and leadership qualities.
2. As siblings they share a special _____ that parents need to _____ and _____.
3. With regard to one another, we are called to:
   a. Romans 12:10 _____ _____
   b. Romans 15:7 _____
   c. 1 Thessalonians 5:11 _____ and

   _____
   d. 1 Thessalonians 5:13 _____ ____ ____ _____
   e. 1 Thessalonians 5:15 _____ _____

4. We did not believe in playing the role of _____ or _____.
5. Learning _____ _____ skills at a young age is very important.

Action Steps: Do as many as you can

What will I do specifically to

1. recognize and encourage each child to pursue their own journey with God?

2. promote and nurture the sibling relationship in my family?

3. avoid the role of referee or counselor?

4. help my children develop conflict resolution skills?

Part II Chapter 11 Time

1. It is impossible to separate our _____ commitments from our _____ of priority.
2. Our children _____ our time.
3. The question is how to _____ and _____?
4. The question is how _____ is _____?
5. My child is a _____ from God that _____ to God and is placed under my _____.
6. Time is a daily _____ that attracts many _____.
7. Time is an _____ trust—when invested wisely—produces _____ treasure.

Action Steps: Do as many as you can.

What will I do specifically to

1. schedule life necessities and exercise time to maintain my physical heath?

2. ensure my work/school/committee time produces a high ROI (return on investment) and low OC (opportunity cost)?

3. schedule "me" time (this is healthy in moderation), couple time, and family time so I can enjoy my friends, my spouse, and my children?

4. not lose sight I am first and foremost an ambassador of Christ and need church fellowship and involvement in my life?

Part II Chapter 12 Stewardship

1. Our _____ and our _____
   on earth are _____ .
2. In order for love to be _____ , it
   must be _____ .
3. Stewardship is the _____ of God's
   _____ .
4. God uses _____ as _____
   for His children.
5. God has fashioned by hand children for you to
   _____ and _____ .
6. By _____ grade my child has lived
   _____ of their expected time in my
   home.
7. My relationship with my child _____
   will determine my relationship with them
   _____ .

Action Steps: Do as many as you can.

What will I do specifically to

1. create a home where stewardship takes place?

2. help each child understand the risk and rewards associated with my freedom of choice?

3. teach each child about their past, their present, and their future with God?

4. ensure your children want to visit with you after they leave home?

Part II Chapter 13 Learning in Joy

1. _____ expectations breed
   _____.

2. Parents need to find _____ in the
   _____.

3. Parents need to discover _____ in
   _____.

4. _____ leads to _____.

5. Parents should be full of _____ and
   _____.

6. Our _____ is in process of becoming
   _____.

7. _____ leads to Joy and Joy leads to
   _____.

Action Steps: Do as many as you can.

What will I do specifically to

1. remember the joy in parenting today and tomorrow?

2. make my home a joyful place to live and visit?

3. express my joy in parenting to others?

4. be joyful always (1 Thess. 5:16)?

Part III Chapter 14 Purposeful Planning

1. God has a wonderful _____ for our lives.
2. The four elements of purposeful planning are
   a. _____
   b. _____
   c. _____
   d. _____

Plot

1. A plot is a greater _____ to be carried out in the future.
2. Name three threats that undermine our objectives:
   a. _____
   b. _____
   c. _____

3. Value a lasting, positive _____ relationship.

Inform

1. _____, _____, _____ and direct each child in the way he/she should go.
2. God has given us
   a. His _____ to instruct
   b. Jesus as a _____ to follow

c. The Holy Spirit to _____ us

Perform

1. _____, _____, and _____ the plan.
2. Remain _____ as circumstances and outside forces change.
3. Stay true to your original _____.
4. It is important that our plot be consistent with _____ and adaptable to the unique _____ and _____ God has placed with each child.

Evaluate

1. Frequent _____ are necessary to see how well our objectives are being met.
2. Be ready to measure, gauge, calculate, _____, and compute your plot.
3. Encourage your _____ to develop the plot so they are more likely to perform the plot.
4. Consistent communication that is _____ and _____ is key.

Action Steps: Do as many as you can.

What will I do specifically to

1. plan for my children's success?

2. understand God's plan for my children?

3. develop my children's mission objectives?

4. establish a lasting, positive sibling relationship?

5. teach my children to value what I value and what God values?

6. do things together as a family?

7. encourage my children to develop the plot?

8. evaluate my children's plot with my spouse?

Part III Chapter 15 Are There Any Guarantees?

1. Many children who grow up in a _____ environment, full of love and joy in the church and the home, choose Jesus as their Lord and Savior.

2. Children have the _____ to be like their parents.

3. The more solid a parent's relationship with _____, their spouse and their children, the more difficult it is for children to choose a different way or direction.

4. We will never _____ spending too much time loving, enjoying, and rearing our children.

5. Don't spend time _____ _____ and being _____ _____.

6. The three pitfalls that lead to regretting your parenting experience are
   a. _____
   b. _____
   c. _____

7. _____ expectations will only lead to disappointment, disillusionment, and discouragement for the parent and child.

8. Love, support, and encouragement lead to _____ and _____.

Action Steps: Do as many as you can.

What will I do specifically to

1. protect my children from turning away from God?

2. make the most of raising my children?

3. make my child Christ-like?

4. maintain a solid relationship with Jesus?

5. allow my children to choose their own areas of interest?

Part III Chapter 16 We Must Learn to Listen!

1. The two questions I should ask my children every night are
   a. _____ best _____
   b. _____ worst _____

2. Family time of sharing must be _____
   and _____.

3. Some issues may require parental _____
   and some issues may require _____.

4. It is _____ and _____ for
   children to listen to their parents best and worst
   parts of the day.

5. The five benefits of family dinner time are
   a. _____
   b. _____
   c. _____
   d. _____
   e. _____

6. Learning how to _____ listen can
   change our relationship with any child.

7. A child's _____ and _____
   are real to them.

8. Listening is not an activity, it is a _____
   _____.

Action Steps: Do as many as you can.

What will I do specifically to

1. listen to my children like our Heavenly Father listens to us?

2. show my children that I enjoy them?

3. help my children work through their feelings and develop a solution to their problems?

4. host family dinner time?

Part III Chapter 17 Parent for Outcomes

1. We have been blessed with an incredible ____ from our Heavenly Father that has some assembly required.
2. Place a high value on _____ and _____ communication.
3. Understand the links between values, _____, accountability and _____.
4. _____ drive _____; commitment determines _____ behavior; and responsible behavior reveals our _____.
5. Priorities help during time of _____.
6. Teach each child the value of _____, the value of _____ and the need to _____ God and others.
7. God has called us to be _____.
8. The greatest ability to lead is our _____ and _____ to serve.

Action Steps: Do as many as you can.

What will I do specifically to

1. improve communication in my household?

2. teach and model values in my household?

3. teach and model stewardship in my household?

4. teach and model leadership in my household?

Part III Chapter 18 This World Is Not Our Home!

1. Children are like treasures in _____ _____.

2. Children can be easily _____ and _____.

3. Our child's first _____ years are critical to their shaping process.

4. We need to raise our children to be _____ about and desire serving Jesus.

5. Our children are _____ treasures from God.

6. _____ glory far outweighs _____ struggles.

7. Fathers, don't lose _____.

8. Mothers, don't _____.

9. We must learn to see our children as _____.

10. _____ made today may reap eternal rewards tomorrow.

11. Our children are treasure God has entrusted to us. We should seek God's guidance and assistance in _____ the treasure back to Him.

Action Steps: Do as many as you can.

What will I do specifically to

1. raise children that are excited about and desire to serve Jesus?

2. see my children as eternal creations?

3. raise my children through the perspective glass of eternity?

4. thank God for the treasure He has entrusted me?

Answer Key to Fill-In-the-Blank Questions

Part I Chapter 1 Marriage Requires

The Foundation of Marriage

1. All marriages face *storms*.
2. *Love* and *respect* are the two primary ingredients for a healthy marriage.
3. A strong foundation is needed both before and after *children*.
4. Children need to see our commitment to *love*, *honor*, and *cherish*.

The Fundamentals of Marriage

1. The four fundamentals of marriage are
   a. *Communication*
   b. *Trust*
   c. *Forgiveness*
   d. *Love*

2. Communication requires both *time* and *effort*.

3. Communication is only as good as it is framed in *love*.
4. We need to *think* before we speak.
5. Marriage is a *trust* relationship.
6. In spite of changes, the *unconditional love* of our mate remains *constant*.
7. The ability to say *I'm sorry* is an absolute must for a healthy marriage.
8. Love is a *choice*.
9. Companionship must be the result of *two becoming one flesh*.
10. Our relationship as husband and wife impacts our *children's* view of marriage.

Part I Chapter 2 Life Hasn't Changed, Roles Have

Church

1. Church is a *vital foundation* of God's kingdom that is being established and used by God for His glory through His people.
2. As our knowledge and understanding change, so do our *roles*.
3. Our family should imitate a *small church*.

Family

1. We must focus our *identity* on our spouse and family.
2. Our primary objective is to enjoy our *relationships* with God and with one another.

3. Relationships are *eternal*, professions are *temporary.*

Work

1. Our business world needs men and women with
    a. *integrity*
    b. *ethics*
    c. *who value what God values*

2. Parents need to choose time with family and *trust* God to honor that commitment.
3. Our calling is to *love* our spouse and to raise our children in the *training* and *instruction* of the Lord.

School

1. When we stop studying and learning, we start *deteriorating.*
2. We must remain *teachable* so the Holy Spirit can mold us and teach us how to best love and respect Christ.
3. Children enjoy learning when parents *participate* in the learning process with them.
4. God has equipped us with a natural parenting intuition and has given us the *Holy Spirit* and His *Word* to help us.
5. Parents must continue to learn so that we will be properly equipped and able to teach and train our family in the way of *righteousness.*

Part I Chapter 3 Divorce from a Kid's Perspective

1. God *hates* divorce.
2. *Children* are often overlooked when a divorce is chosen.
3. Divorce is the *equivalent* to a death in the family.
4. Divorce is a breach of trust that hampers the parent–child *relationship*.
5. Divorce destroys a child's *basic need* for a sense of belonging.
6. Children of divorced parents need a solid *church* youth group.
7. Divorced parents need a solid *Bible-based* support group.
8. Children need to see Mom and Dad in love with each other and *serving Jesus* together.
9. No marriage is beyond *repair*, for in Christ Jesus, all things are possible.
10. Glad to be a dad and calm to be a mom begin with *happy* to be a husband and *joyous* to be a wife.

Part II Chapter 4 Self-Control

1. The first goal of parenting is to have *ignorance* give way to *understanding*; and *disobedience* give way to *obedience*.
2. Children learn *acceptable* behavior by what they are *taught*.
3. God has given me His *Word* to communicate what is *acceptable* behavior for me.

4. God has given me His *Spirit* to dwell within me and to remind me of my commitment to *obedience*.
5. As I allow God's Spirit to fill me, I develop the fruit of *self-control* and am able to say no to *unrighteousness* and yes to *godliness*.
6. The more *self-control* I develop in my life, the more *self-control* I can help my child develop in his/her life.
7. Catch your children doing things *right*!

Part II Chapter 5 Incarnation

1. Young children like to *model* their parents' *behavior*.
2. As a Christian, I am called to *imitate* the behavior of *Jesus*.
3. Disciple means *"one who follows."*
4. We can *relate* to Jesus because He can *relate* to us.
5. As parents, we need to become *servant leaders* to our children.
6. As parents, we need to become *role models* to our children.
7. As parents, we need to *meet* our children at their level of *growth*.

Part II Chapter 6 Security and Trust

1. As my *trust* increases, so does my *security* and *peace* increase.
2. Children are born into this world with a natural sense of *trust*.

3. By adulthood, many people have less *trust* and *security* in their lives.
4. Parents also have *security* needs.
5. A *relationship* with Jesus Christ is the only *relationship* that will provide constant *peace* and *security* without fail.
6. We should be striving for *dependence* instead of *independence*.
7. We must make our home a place of *security* and *trust* for our family.

Part II Chapter 7 Love

1. Parents need to show *unconditional* love and *acceptance* to their children.
2. Choosing to love is a *natural* behavior for a child.
3. Choosing to love is a *learned* behavior for an adult.
4. God is *love*.
5. *Conditional* love teaches our children that *results* are more important than effort.
6. *Conditional* love teaches our children that *accomplishment* is more important than *character*.
7. *Parents* can learn much about love by watching their *children*.

Part II Chapter 8 Image

1. Mankind alone is *created* in the *image* of God.
2. Mankind is still in the *image* of God after the *fall*.
3. *Image* goes much deeper than *physical* resemblance.

4. Our *spiritual* nature desires for us to *display* the image of God.

5. As we *display* the image of God, we become *conformed* to the image of Christ.

6. Children learn through *observation*.

7. As parents we are *mediators*.

Part II Chapter 9 Discipline and Repentance

1. God has blessed my child with a *wonderful* and *unique* personality.

2. Parents need to *train* each child to *know* the *Master's* will.

3. Start with a *firm* line of discipline during the *early* years.

4. Discipline over *issues* that matter to *God*.

5. Parents need to take the *time* necessary to *administer* proper discipline.

6. Discipline because you *love* the child and desire to *communicate* acceptable behavior.

7. Teaching *discipline* encompasses far more than *punishment*.

Part II Chapter 10 One Another

1. Each child is *uniquely* gifted with talents, personalities and leadership qualities.

2. As siblings they share a special *bond* that parents need to *promote* and *nurture*.

3. With regard to one another, we are called to:

     a.   Romans 12:10 *be devoted*

     b.   Romans 15:7 *accept*

     c.   1 Thessalonians 5:11 *encourage* and *build-up*

     d.   1 Thessalonians 5:13 *live in peace with*

     e.   1 Thessalonians 5:15 *be kind*

4.   We did not believe in playing the role of *referee* or *counselor*.

5.   Learning *conflict resolution* skills at a young age is very important.

Part II Chapter 11 Time

1.   It is impossible to separate our *time* commitments from our *order* of priority.

2.   Our children *require* our time.

3.   The question is how to *balance* and *prioritize?*

4.   The question is how *much* is *enough?*

5.   My child is a *gift* from God that *belongs* to God and is placed under my *care*.

6.   Time is a daily *treasure* that attracts many *robbers*.

7.   Time is an *earthly* trust—when invested wisely—produces *eternal* treasure.

Part II Chapter 12 Stewardship

1.   Our *time* and our *treasures* on earth are *temporary*.

2.   In order for love to be *real,* it must be *free*.

3.   Stewardship is the *management* of God's *resources*.

4.   God uses *parents* as *stewards* for His children.

5. God has fashioned by hand children for you to *enjoy* and *teach*.
6. By *first* grade, my child has lived *one-third* of their expected time in my home.
7. My relationship with my child *today* will determine my relationship with them *tomorrow*.

Part II Chapter 13 Learning in Joy

1. *Exciting* expectations breed *joy*.
2. Parents need to find *joy* in the *journey*.
3. Parents need to discover *learning* in *joy*.
4. *Joy* leads to *praise*.
5. Parents should be full of *joy* and *praise*.
6. Our *joy* is in process of becoming *complete*.
7. *Learning* leads to joy and joy leads to *learning*.

Part III Chapter 14 Purposeful Planning

1. God has a wonderful *plan* for our lives.
2. The four elements of purposeful planning are
   a. *plot*
   b. *inform*
   c. *perform*
   d. *evaluate*

Plot

1. A plot is a greater *purpose* to be carried out in the future.

2. Name three threats that undermine our objectives:
    a. *sinful nature*
    b. *fiery darts from the evil one*
    c. *love of the world*

3. Value a lasting, positive *sibling* relationship.

Inform

1. *prepare, explain, instruct,* and direct each child in the way he/she should go.
2. God has given us:
    a. His *Word* to instruct
    b. Jesus as a *model* to follow
    c. The Holy Spirit to *help* us

Perform

1. *implement, execute,* and *complete* the plan.
2. Remain *flexible* as circumstances and outside forces change.
3. Stay true to your original *objective.*
4. It is important that our plot be consistent with *scripture* and adaptable to the unique *gifts* and *desires* God has placed with each child.

Evaluate

1. Frequent *performance evaluations* are necessary to see how well our objectives are being met.

2. Be ready to measure, gauge, calculate, *determine*, and compute your plot.
3. Encourage your *children* to develop the plot so they are more likely to perform the plot.
4. Consistent communication that is *planned* and *purposeful* is key.

Part III Chapter 15 Are There Any Guarantees?

1. Many children who grow up in a *Christian* environment, full of love and joy in the church and the home, choose Jesus as their Lord and Savior.
2. Children have the *tendency* to be like their parents.
3. The more solid a parent's relationship with *Jesus*, their spouse, and their children, the more difficult it is for children to choose a different way or direction.
4. We will never *regret* spending too much time loving, enjoying, and rearing our children.
5. Don't spend time *stressing out* and being *too busy.*
6. The three pitfalls that lead to regretting your parenting experience are
   a. *trying to do it all*
   b. *poor planning*
   c. *ignoring/fighting the surprises life gives us*

7. *Unnecessary* expectations will only lead to disappointment, disillusionment, and discouragement for the parent and child.

8. Love, support, and encouragement lead to *acceptance* and *joy*.

Part III Chapter 16 We Must Learn to Listen!

1. The two questions you should ask your children every night are
   a. *What is the* best *thing that happened to you today?*
   b. *What is the* worst *thing that happened to you today?*

2. Family time of sharing must be *respected* and *open*.
3. Some issues may require parental *privacy* and some issues may require *discipline*.
4. It is *important* and *fun* for children to listen to their parents' best and worst parts of the day.
5. The five benefits of family dinner time are
   a. *teachable moments for the children*
   b. *opportunities for family prayer*
   c. *further discussions for Mom and Dad*
   d. *a growing sense of family*
   e. *teammates committed to relational growth and common objectives*

6. Learning how to *actively* listen can change our relationship with any child.
7. A child's *fears* and *concerns* are real to them.
8. Listening is not an activity, it is a *way of life*.

Part III Chapter 17 Parent for Outcomes

1. We have been blessed with an incredible *gift* from our Heavenly Father that has some assembly required.
2. Place a high value on *open* and *honest* communication.
3. Understand the links between values, *behavior*, accountability and *consequences*.
4. *Values* drive c*ommitment*; commitment determines *responsible* behavior; and responsible behavior reveals our *testimony*.
5. Priorities help during time of *conflict*.
6. Teach each child the value of *stewardship*, the value of *surrendering* and the need to *serve* God and others.
7. God has called us to be *leaders*.
8. The greatest ability to lead is our *availability* and *willingness* to serve.

Part III Chapter 18 This World Is Not Our Home!

1. Children are like treasures in *jars of clay*.
2. Children can be easily *molded* and *shaped*.
3. Our child's first *twelve* years are critical to their shaping process.
4. We need to raise our children to be *excited* about and desire serving Jesus.
5. Our children are *eternal* treasures from God.
6. *Eternal* glory far outweighs *temporary* struggles.

7. Fathers, don't lose *heart.*
8. Mothers, don't *despair.*
9. We must learn to see our children as *eternal creations.*
10. *Sacrifices* made today may reap eternal rewards tomorrow.
11. Our children are treasures God has entrusted to us. We should seek God's guidance and assistance in *presenting* the treasure back to Him.

CPSIA information can be obtained
at www.ICGtesting.com
Printed in the USA
FFHW020206200119
50219168-55202FF